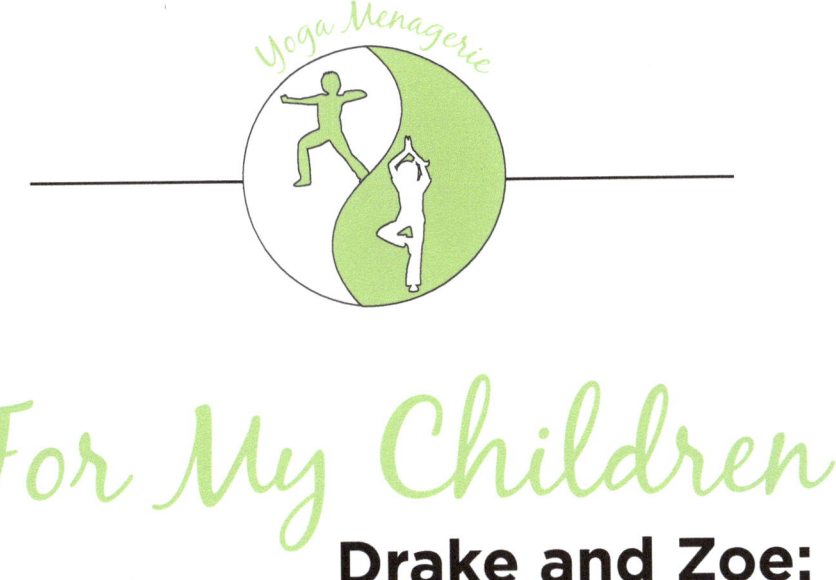

Yoga Menagerie

For My Children

Drake and Zoe;

May You Always Follow Your Flow

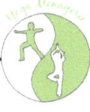

Yoga Menagerie's

POSITIVE AFFIRMATION RE'FLEX'IONS

Book Two

BY: VICTORIA FISHMAN
ILLUSTRATED BY: MORGAN KELLER

Positive Affirmations are a technique used to focus the mind on a specific goal in a positive and empowering way. Repeating Positive Affirmations daily helps to assist in increasing the ability to think positively. The words in the affirmation trigger the mind into positive action and act as a tool for shedding limiting thought patterns. Saying Positive Affirmations are a way to experience having a positive outlook.

The following Positive Affirmation Flows are designed to combine Positive Affirmations with Vinyasa (flow) Yoga. The Positive Affirmation Flows are done by saying the affirmations; (either out loud or to yourself), while you are performing the yoga poses in the flow. The Positive Affirmation Flows help to bring improvements to your physical and mental health and assist in creating a positive attitude. To be most effective these affirmations should always be said with; focus, interest, intent, desire and sincerity.

This book contains a amazing alphabetized picture glossary to help you learn and explain the poses. It also includes a special section for Yoga Journaling so everyone can chart their progress and record their experiences.

This book also contains a special chapter focusing on combining character building concepts with yoga. These sequences are inspired by the yamas and niyamas of Patanjali's Eight Fold Path. They explore concepts referring to social and ethical guidelines and help to develop qualities that promote living positively.

The Adventure Guide

POSITIVE AFFIRMATION RE'FLEX'IONS (BOOK 2)

POSITIVE AFFIRMATION RE'FLEX'IONS

Chapter One

POSITIVE AFFIRMATION *1*

I am bright and vibrant like the sun;
A beautiful star shining on everyone.

Sun
Star

I am amazing, kind and true;
But I'm a mighty warrior too.

Open Hero
Warrior 1

I soar high above the rest;
I am strong enough for any test.

Bird
Mountain

*This poem can be done on one side and then repeated using the opposite side.

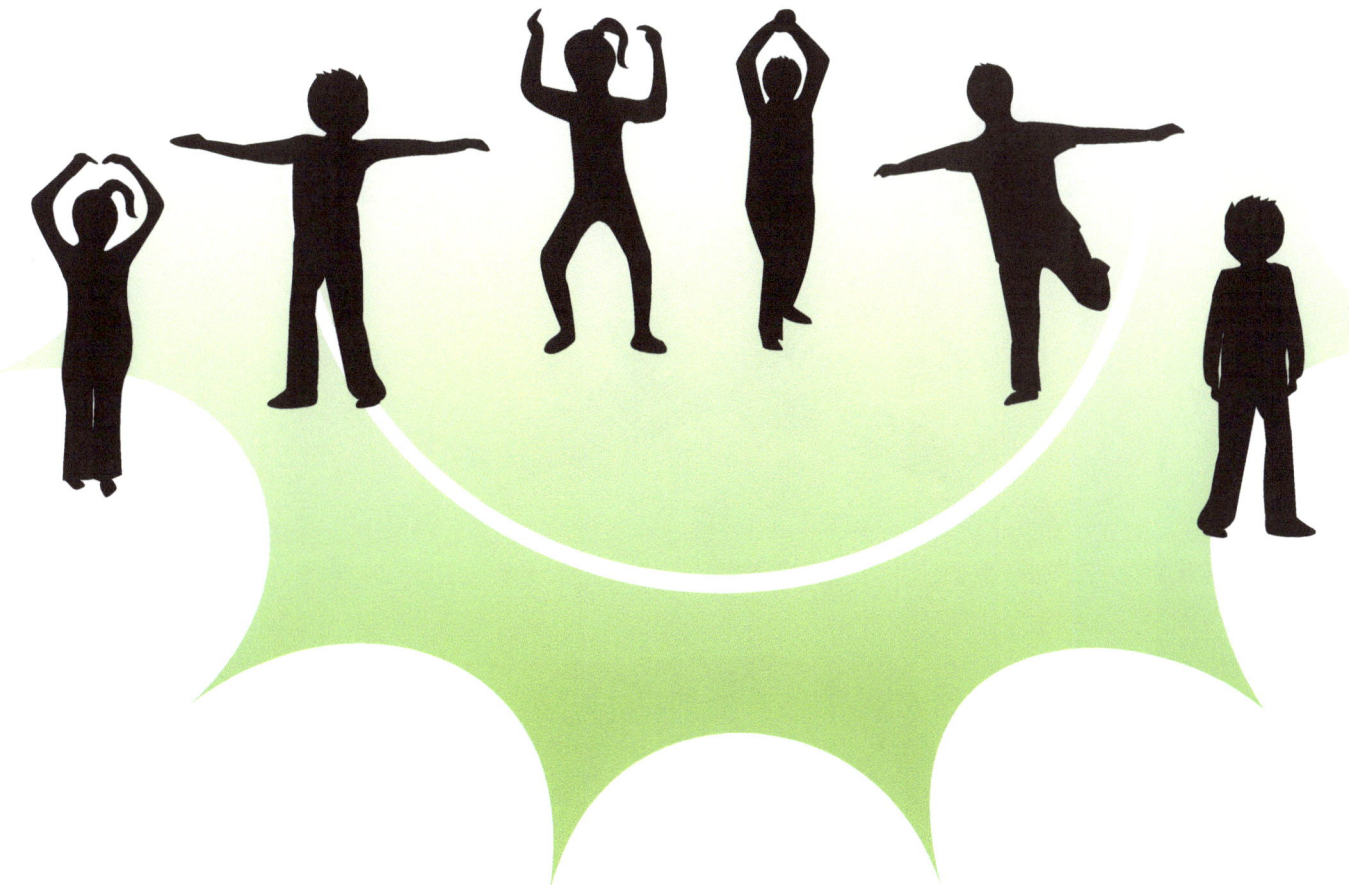

POSITIVE AFFIRMATION 2

I am intelligent like a wise owl;
Focused like when he's on the prowl.

Owl – Right
Owl – Left

I am as strong as a grizzly bear;
And I'm always flexible and fair.

Open To Bear
Reach To Center

I am responsible like
my friend the turtle;
And I can carry myself
over any hurdle.

Turtle

Tuck Head Down

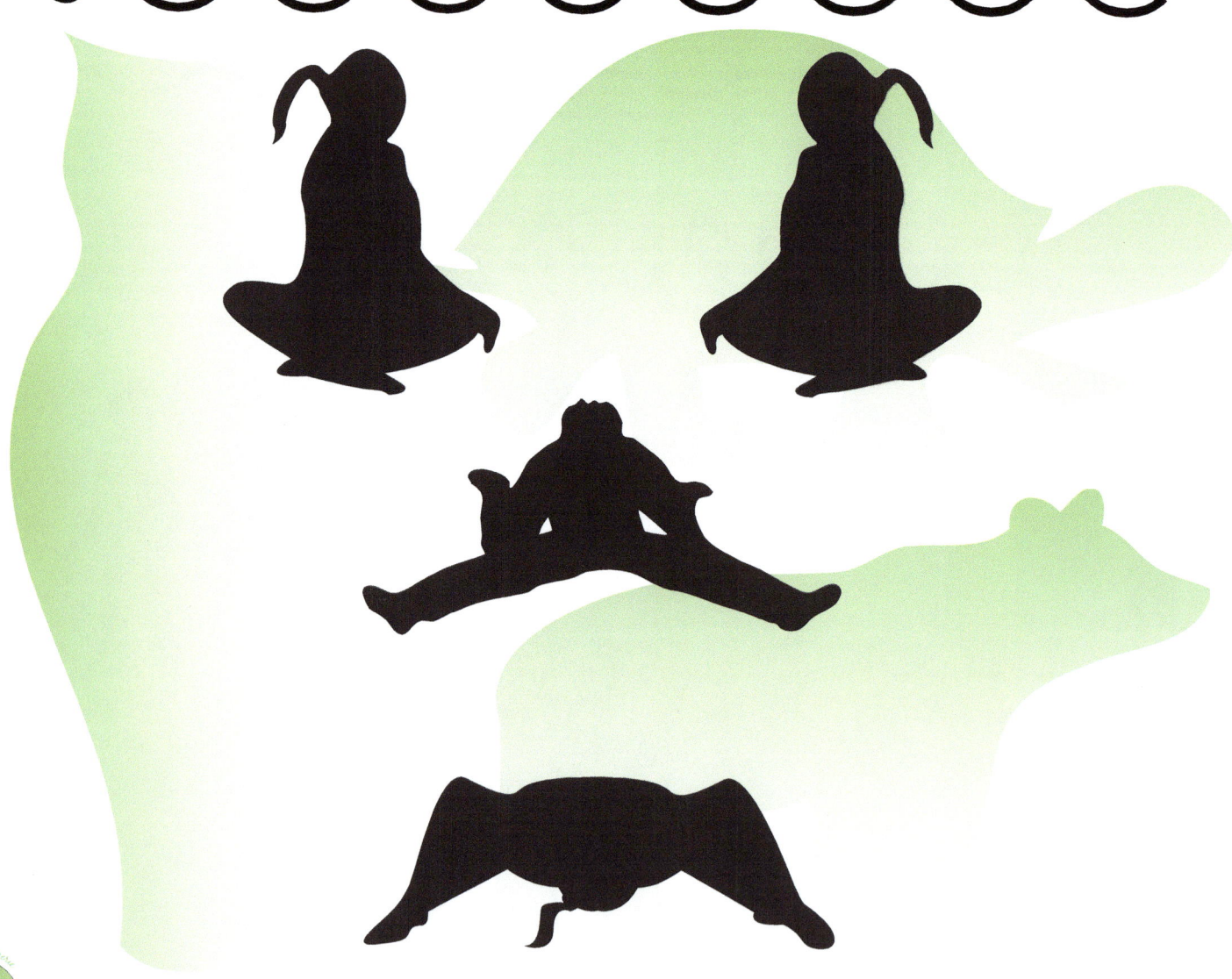

POSITIVE AFFIRMATION 3

I light up the world like the moon does at night;
I am confident that I will know what is right.

I'm like a peacock sure and proud;
And I'm not afraid to say it loud.

I am clever and bold like a fox;
I am always ready when opportunity knocks.

I am alert and aware of everything around me;
I am content that all things are as they should be.

*This poem can be done on one side and then repeated using the opposite side.

Crescent Moon – Left
Crescent Moon – Right

Peacock
Lift arms up

Down Dog

Mountain
Star

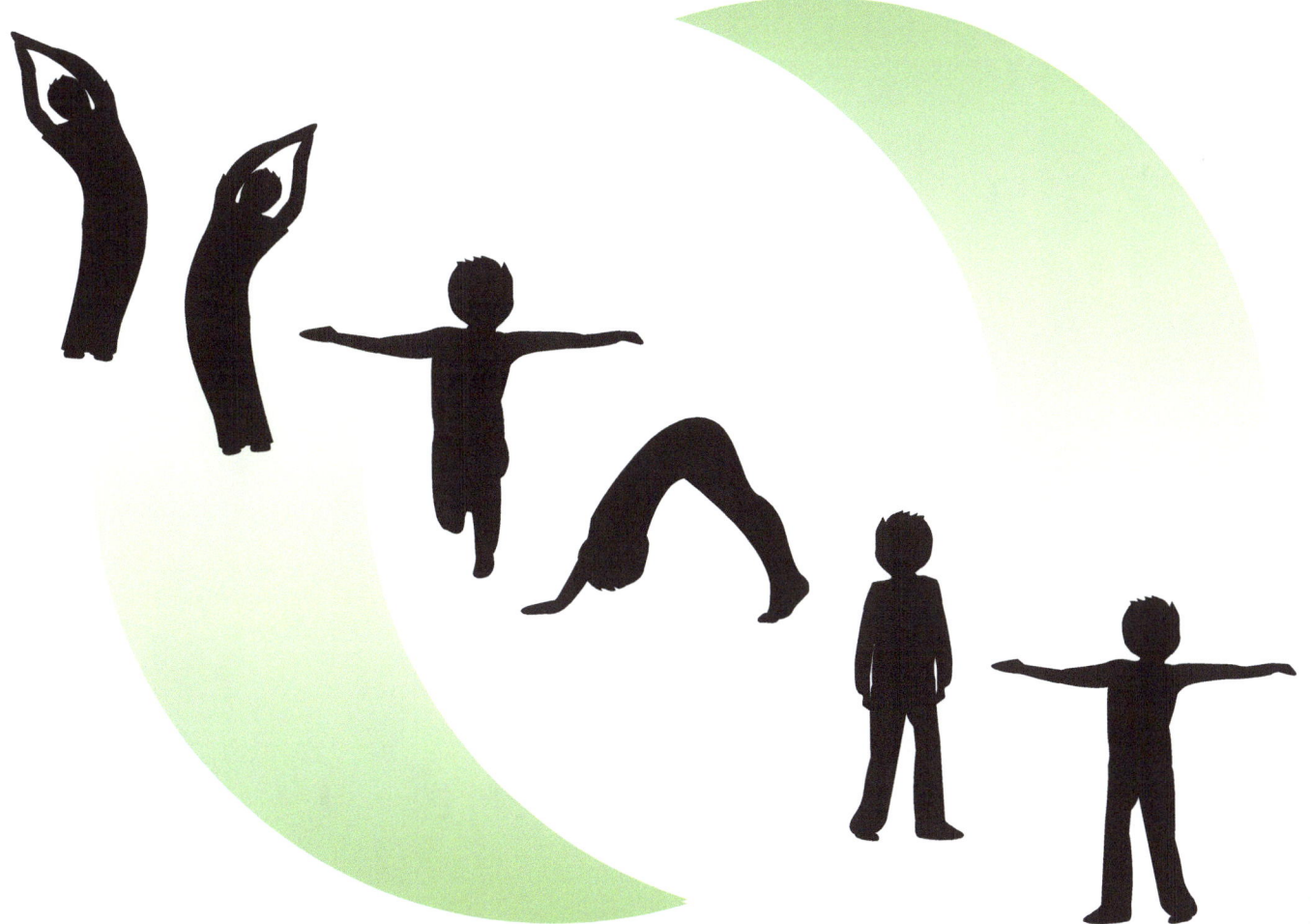

POSITIVE AFFIRMATION 4

I am as sweet as a honey bee;   *Bee 1*
I can share the love inside of me.   *Bee 2*

I am as quiet as a little cat;   *Cat Tilt Up*
I find peace in silence like that.   *Cat Tilt Down*

I am grounded just like a tiny seed;   *Squat*
I feel the earth give me all my needs; *Extend Arms Out*

I can become anything if only I try;   *Mountain*
With my roots in the ground, I reach for the sky.   *Tree*

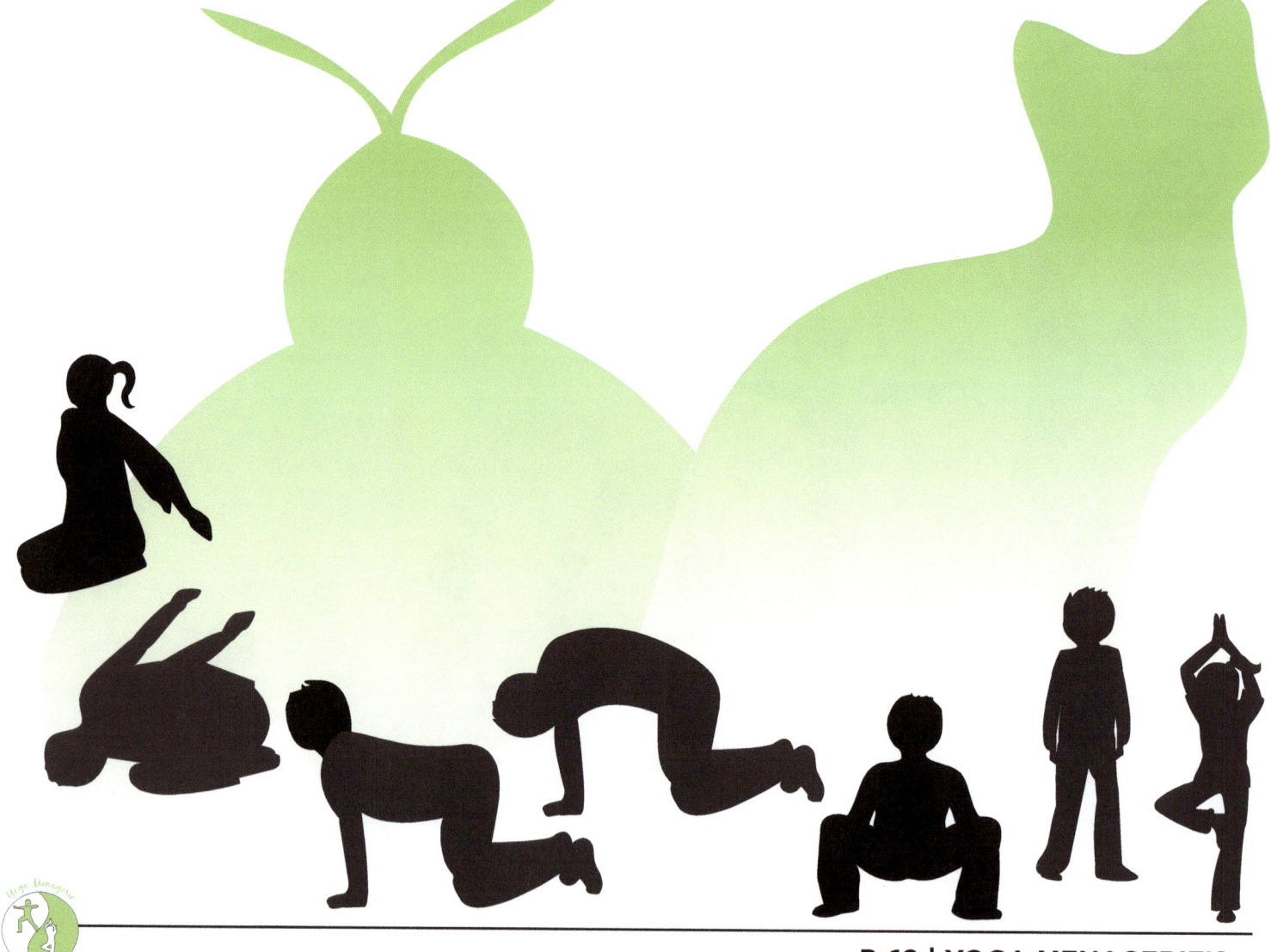

POSITIVE AFFIRMATION 5

I am a rock solid and strong;   *Rock*
I know exactly where I belong.

I am honest, fair and true;   *Down Dog*
Just like a dog I'm loyal too.

I can remember like an elephant;   *Elephant*
So I've only used words that I really meant.

Just like an eagle I let my spirit soar;   *Eagle*
The whole world is ready for me to explore

*This poem can be done on one side and then repeated using the opposite side.

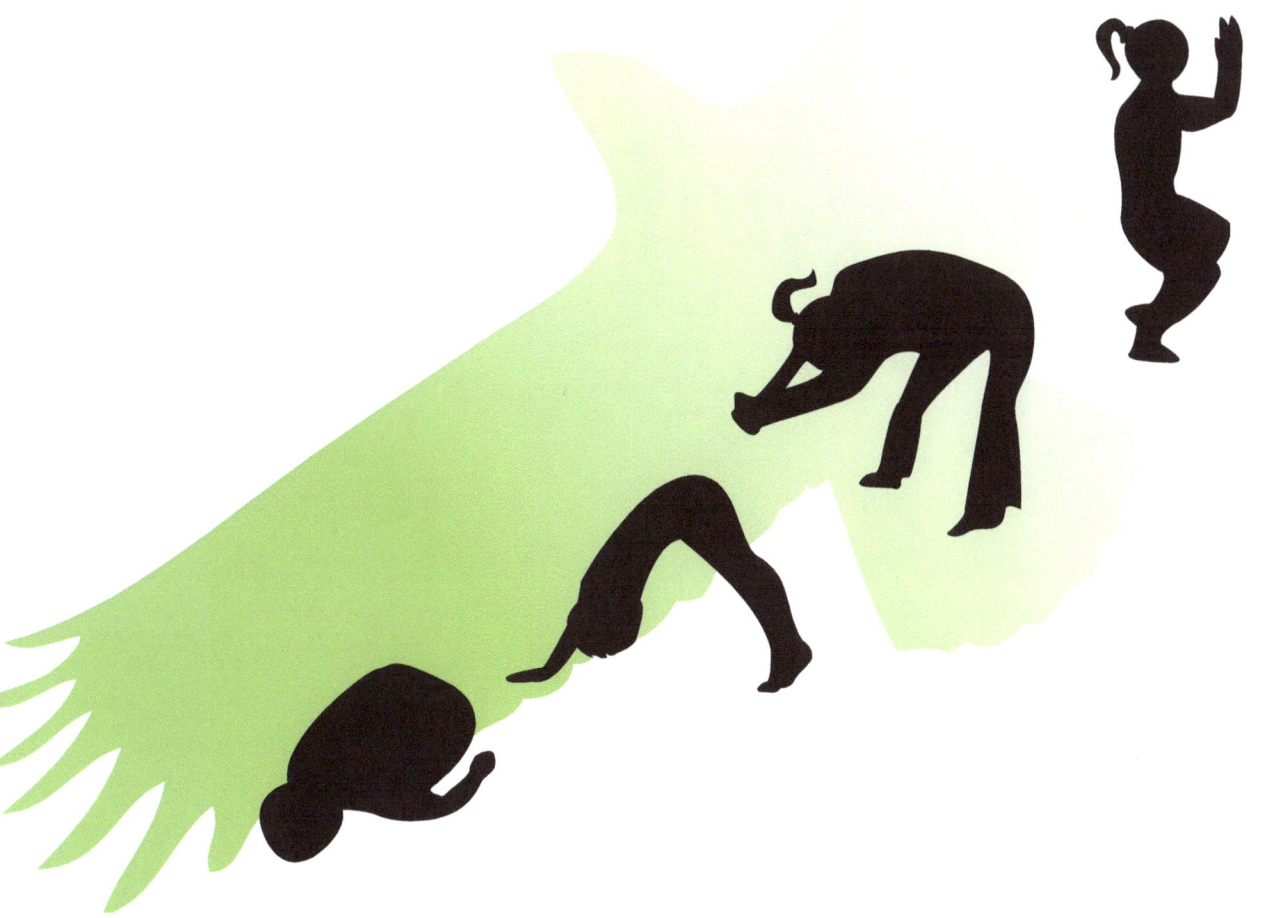

POSITIVE AFFIRMATION 6

I am a butterfly graceful and free;   *Butterfly*
I can soar wherever I want to be.

I can be peaceful like the deer;   *Deer – Right*
Because I know I can be present here.   *Deer – Left*

I am as flexible as a rainbow;   *Rainbow*
Accepting change helps me let go.

I can let go of all my fears;   *Lion 1*
With lion I feel my courage near.   *Lion 2*

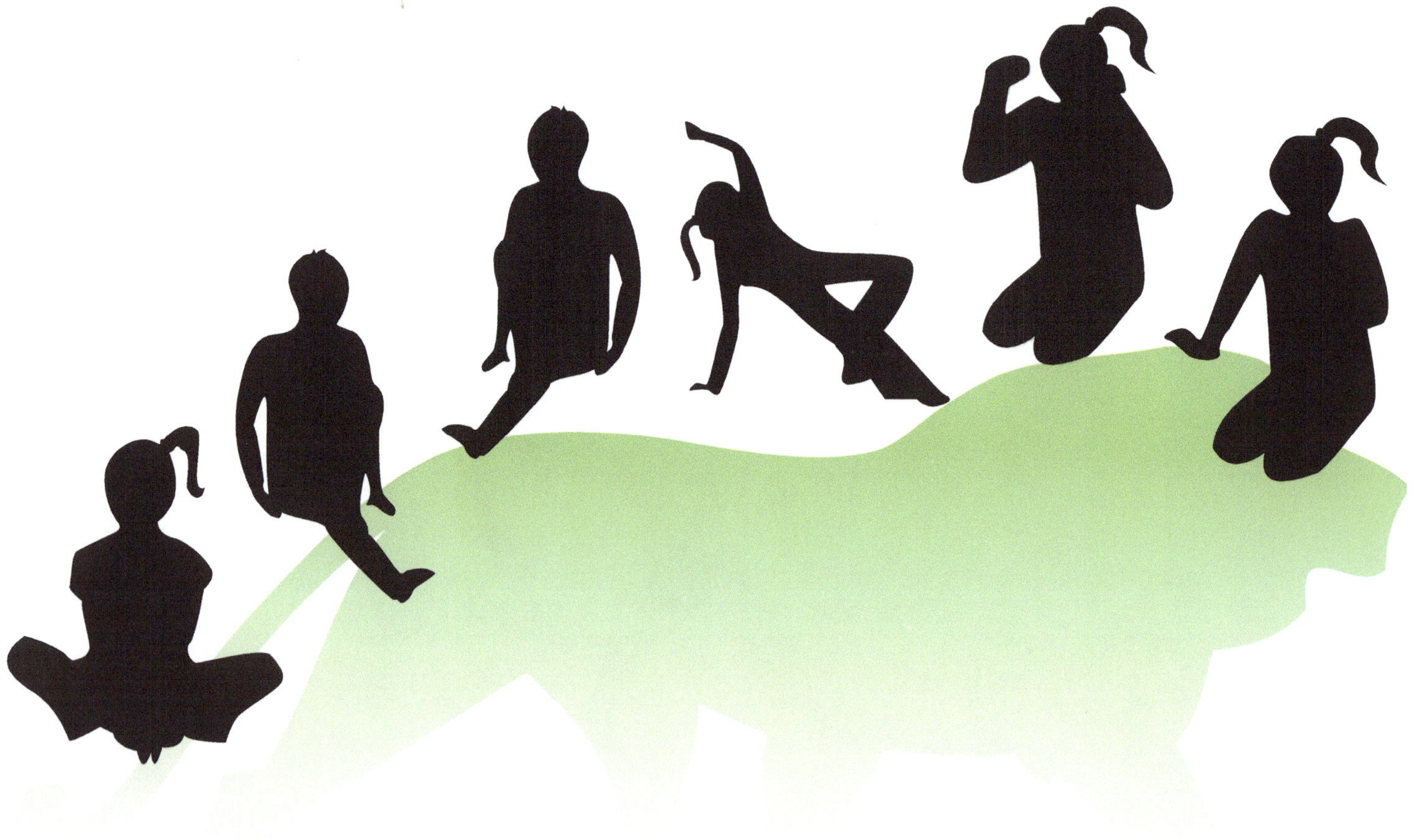

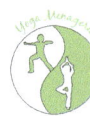

POSITIVE AFFIRMATION 7

I am bright and dazzling like the moon;
And I shine like the sun up in the sky at noon.

I sparkle like a twinkling star;
I share my light with those near and far.

I can hike up tall mountains, or a volcano;
Pick anywhere, choose a direction and GO!

Crescent moon – Right
Sun

Star
Archer - Right

Mountain – Volcano
Circle Around - Mt

*This poem can be done on one side and then repeated using the opposite side.

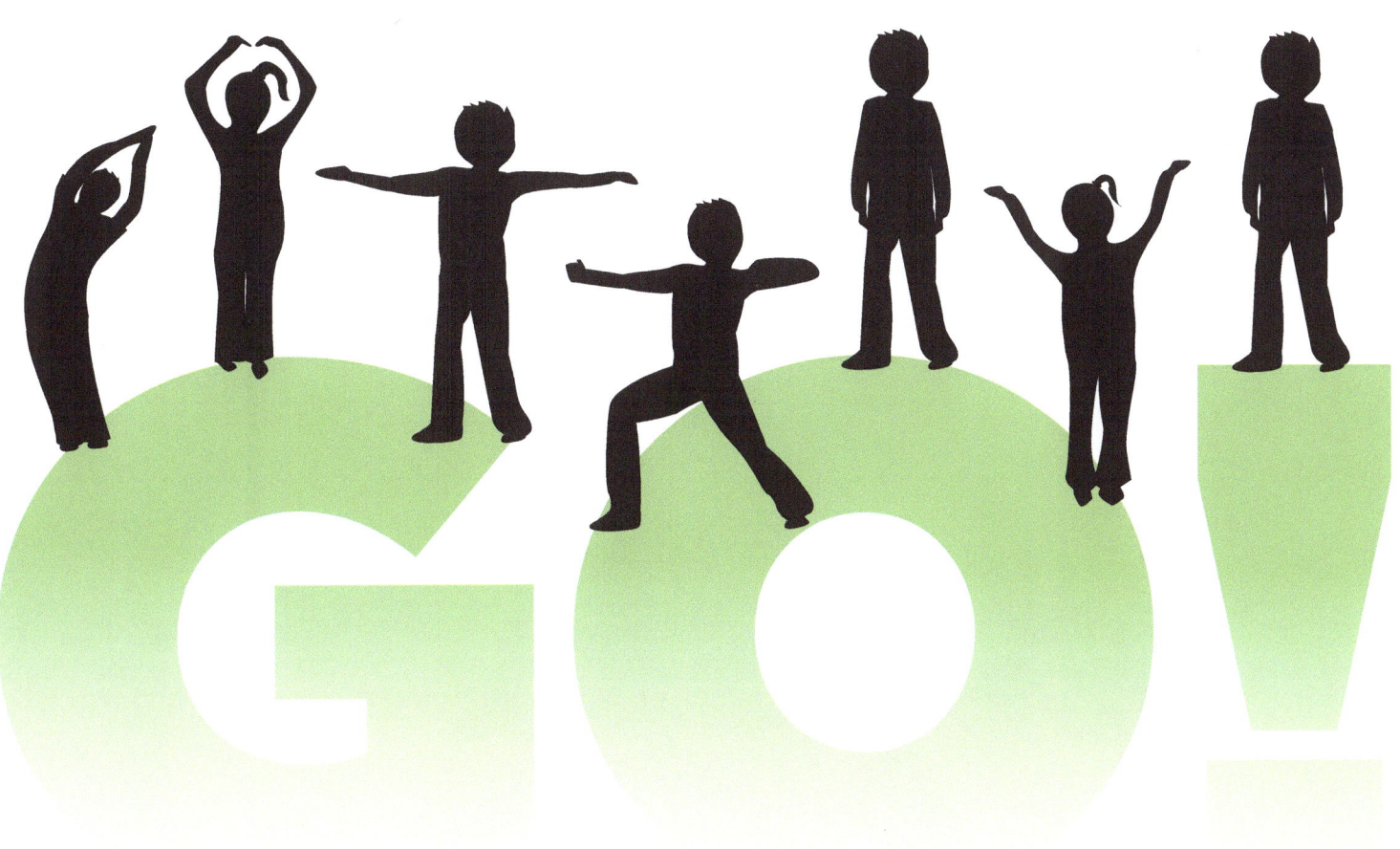

POSITIVE AFFIRMATION 8

I can surf on the waves and sail on the tide;   *Warrior 2*
Whatever I do – I do it with pride.   *Warrior 1*

I can soar up in a plane, balloon or jet,   *Bird – Right*
No matter what I do - I'm my best bet.   *Bird – Left*

I can go all around the Earth;   *Open Hero*
But I look inside to find my true worth.   *Washing Machine*

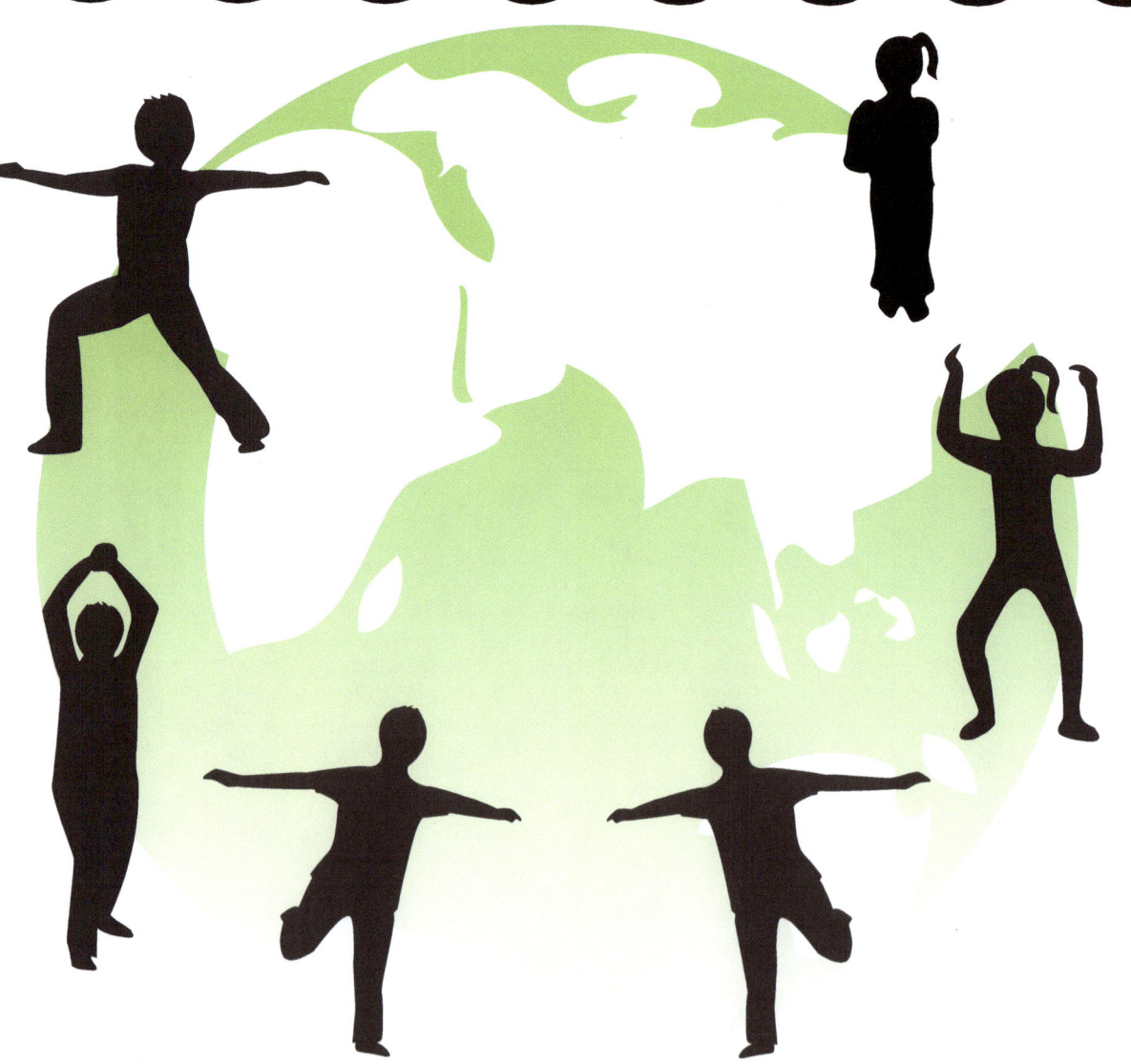

POSITIVE AFFIRMATION 9

I am unique as a butterfly's wings;   *Butterfly*
I open my heart and let it sing.   *Bear*

I am as distinct as a turtle's shell;   *Turtle*
I am extraordinary as well.

I am an exceptional find;   *Owl – Right*
I am the only one of my kind.   *Owl – Left*

I am special like a little seed;   *Flower*
Watch me bloom and grow into me.

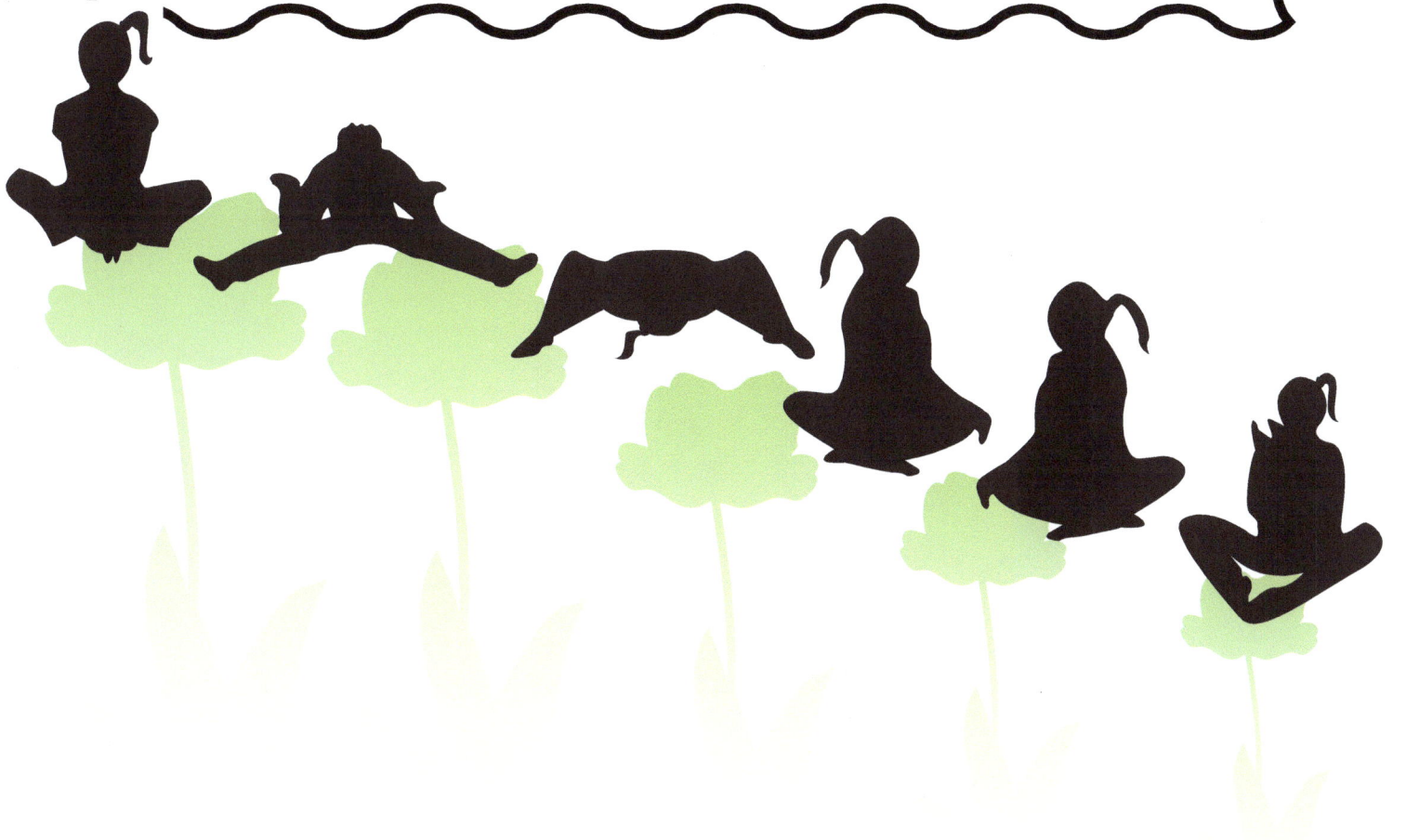

POSITIVE AFFIRMATION *10*

With my body I take great care;   *Bear*
So I can be as strong as a bear.

I always try to eat what's right;   *Owl - Right*
And keep my dreams & goals in sight.   *Owl - Left*

Things that I eat give me fuel to run;   *Deer - Right*
So like a deer I can play and have fun.   *Deer - Left*

I work hard to be really healthy;   *Down Dog*
So like a fox, I can be stealthy.

I work hard each and everyday   *Triangle*
To make my body feel Okay!   *Mountain*

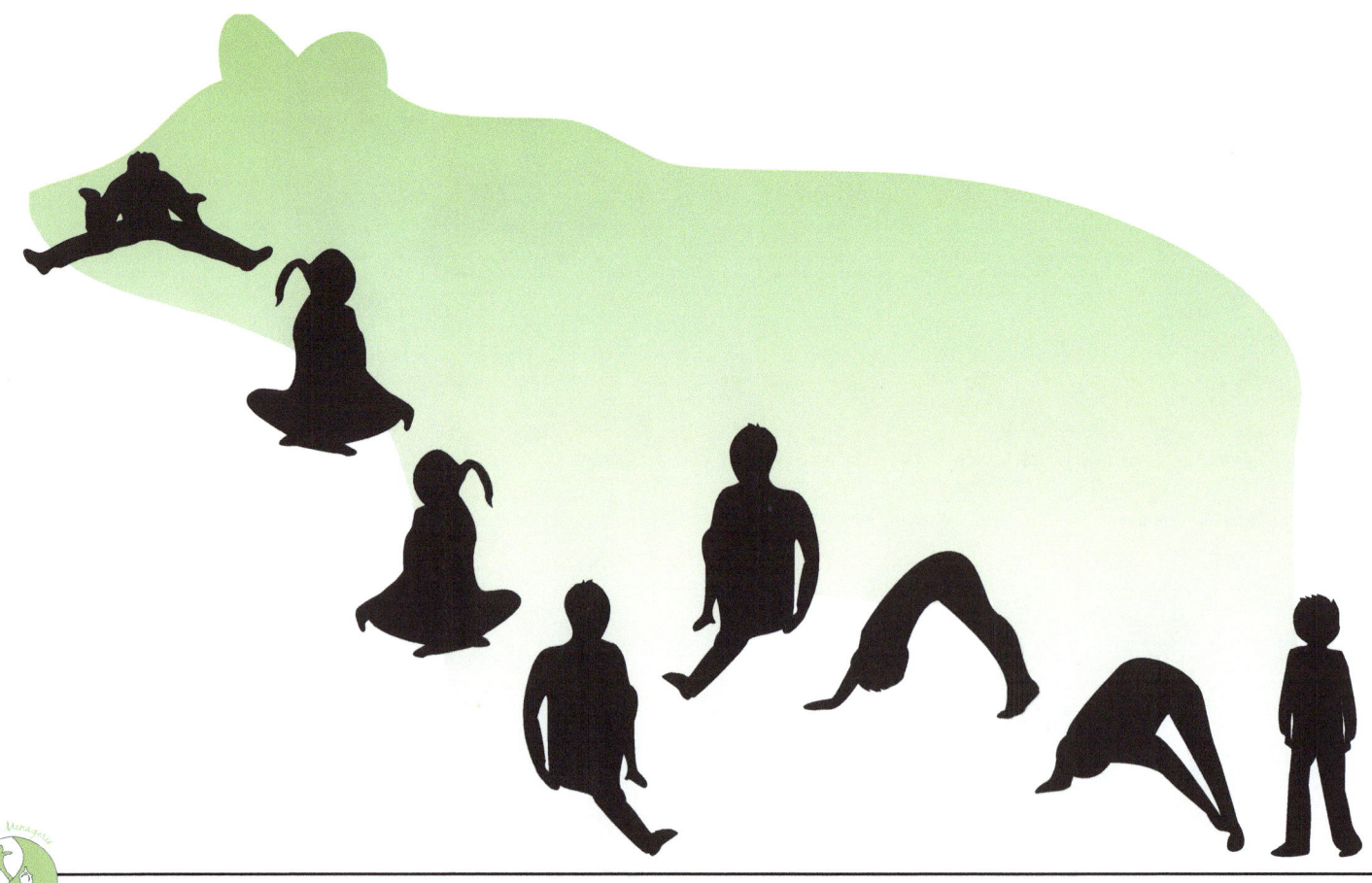

POSITIVE AFFIRMATION *11*

I am clever and cunning like a snake;   *Cobra*
I put great effort into everything I make.
I am strong and flexible like a shark;   *Shark*
And I'm not afraid to make my mark.
Like a swan I'm graceful and sleek;   *Swan*
And I act strong when I feel weak.
I keep on moving like the fish;   *Fish*
And I'll never stop til I get my wish.
When I come to a place that's hard to cross;
I build myself a bridge across.   *Bridge*

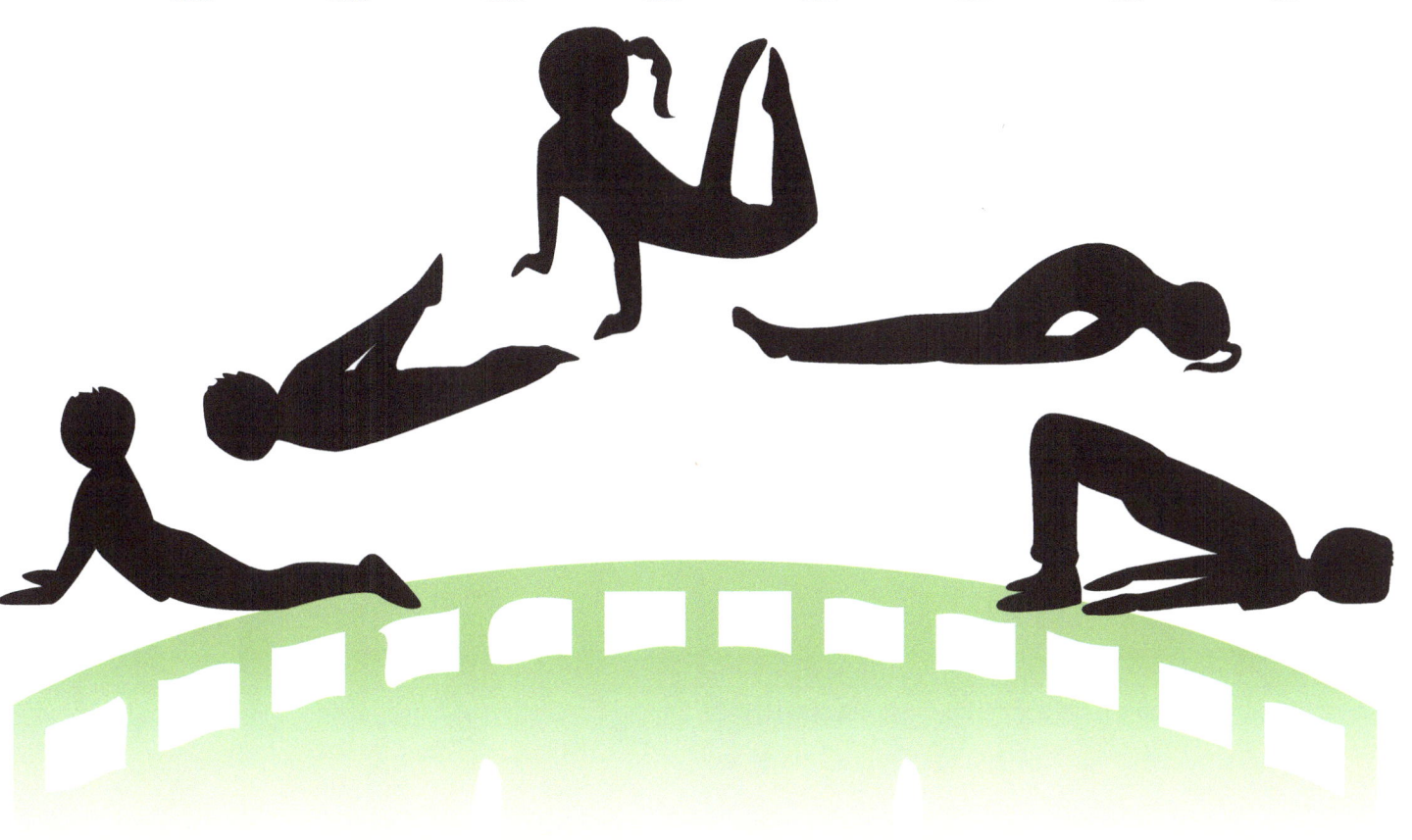

POSITIVE AFFIRMATION *12*

I believe in myself, I'm fearless & true;	*Warrior 2*
I am bold and strong like a warrior too.	*Warrior 3*
I am determined, I will never stop;	*Archer*
Like an archer, I always take my shot.	
I reach for the stars up in the sky;	*Star*
Everything I do - I give it my best try.	
I have confidence in the things I do;	*Warrior 1*
And I always let my true self through.	
I can soar up like a little bird;	*Bird*
And let my inner voice be heard.	

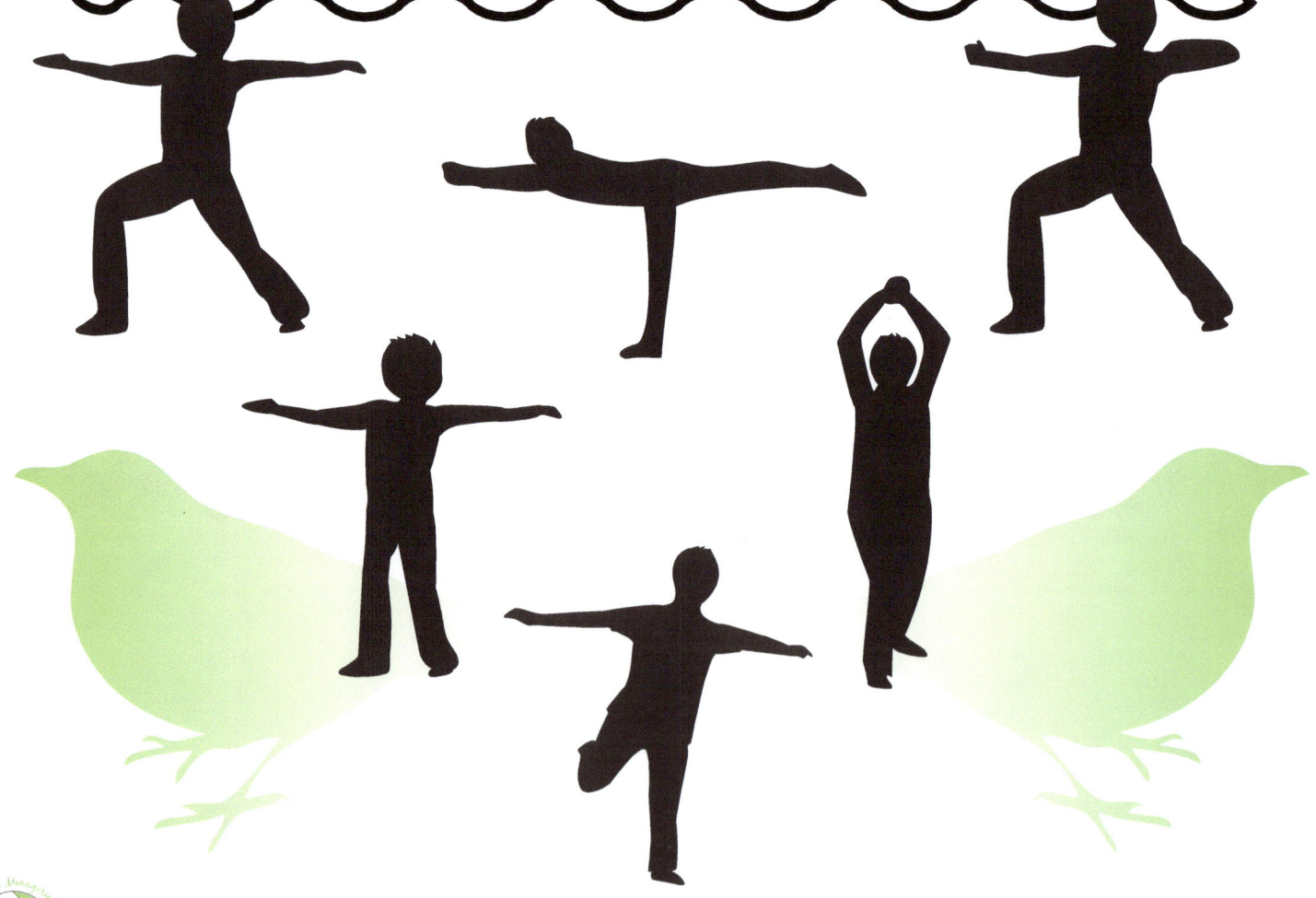

POSITIVE AFFIRMATION *13*

I open my heart so I can set free;
All of the love inside of me.

Archer
Star

I open my eyes so I can see;
What the world is showing me.

Lion 1
Lion 2

I can focus and simply be;
I open my mind and think clearly.

Mountain
Volcano

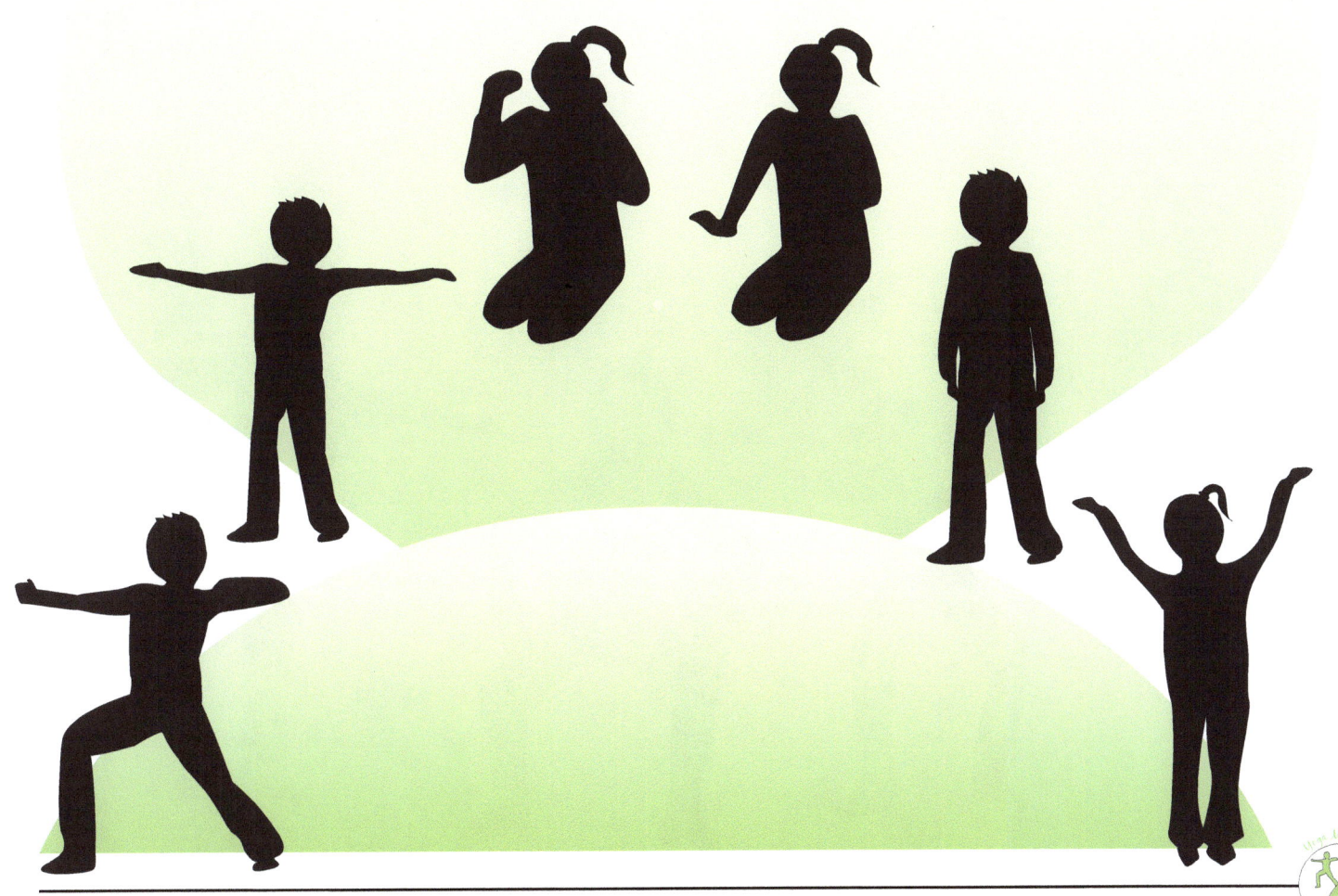

POSITIVE AFFIRMATION *14*

I am sure-footed like a flamingo;   *Flamingo*
I trust in myself and go with the flow.

I have the strength of a horse;   *Horse*
I am determined to follow my course.

Like a gorilla I'm smart and resourceful;   *Gorilla*
I never give up and am always hopeful.

I never dwell on things that have occurred;   *Bird*
I move on and fly just like a bird.

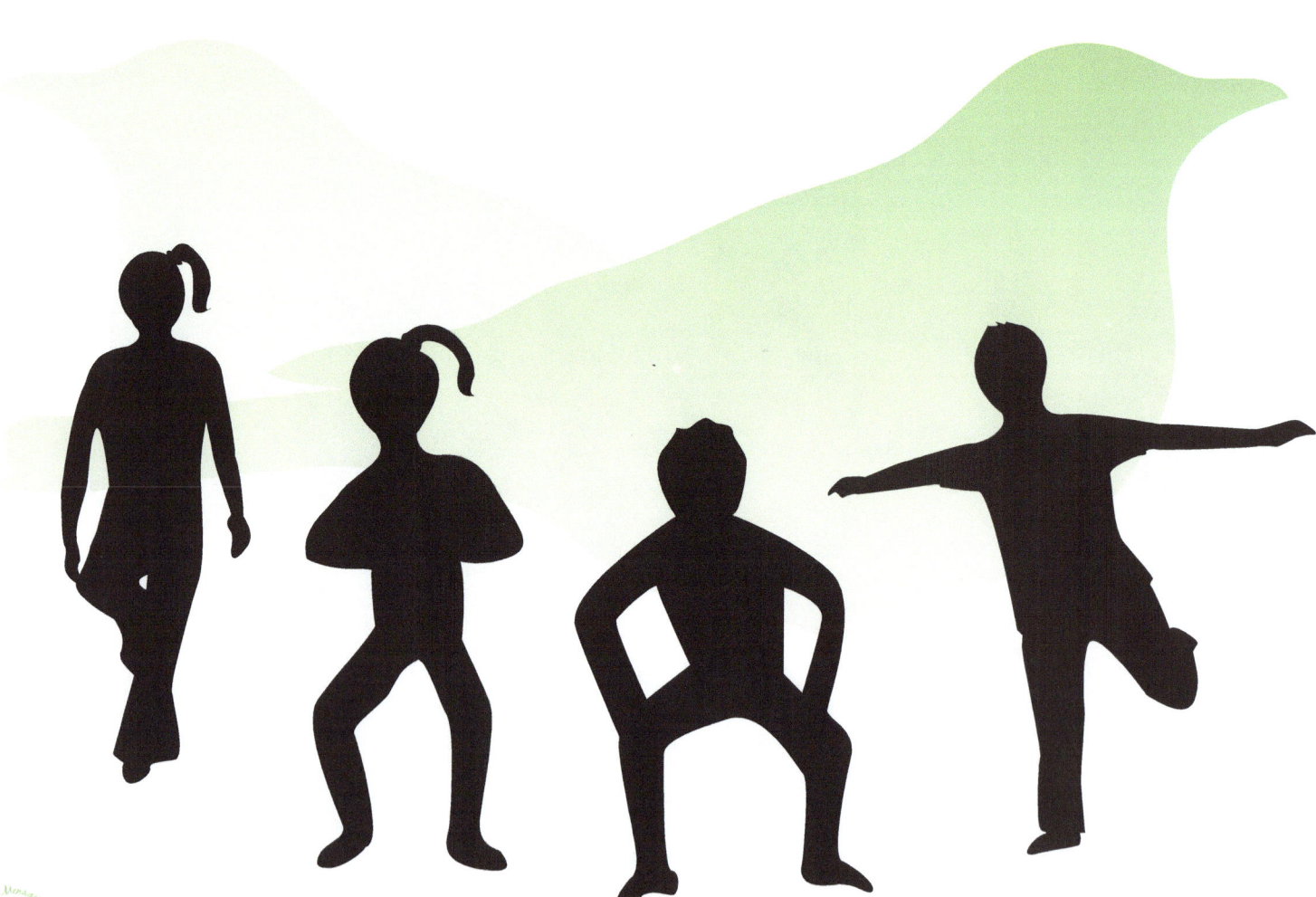

POSITIVE AFFIRMATION *15*

I am kind and gentle like a deer;   *Deer- Right*
I have no trouble overcoming fear.   *Deer- Left*

Flying like a butterfly seeking inspiration;   *Butterfly*
I am moving on a pathway of transformation.

Like an armadillo I protect my boundaries;   *Armadillo*
I know it is myself, I must appease.

No matter the path I'm always persistent;   *Spider*
Like a spider, my work is consistent.

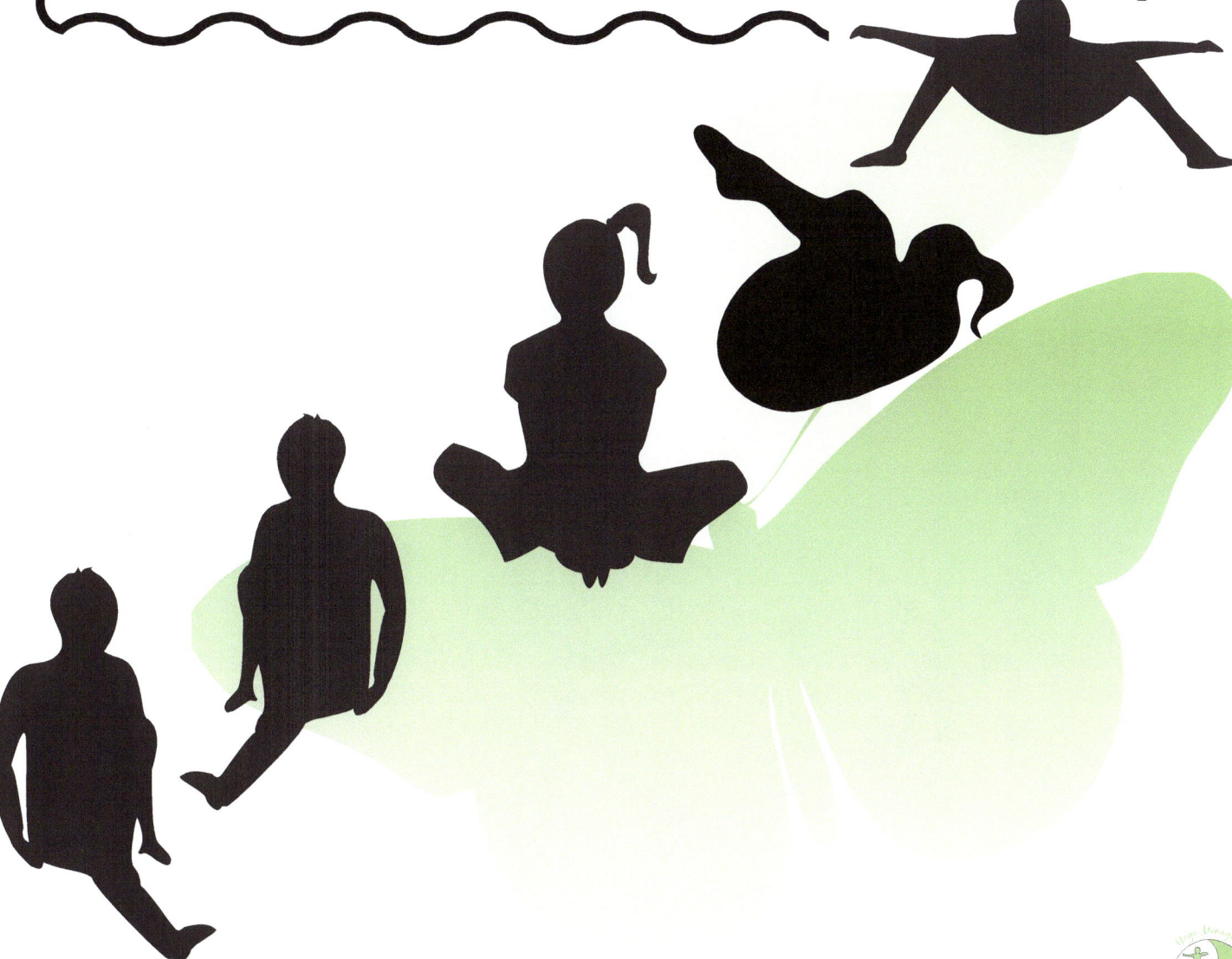

POSITIVE AFFIRMATION *16*

I can move in any direction like a hummingbird;   *Bird*
Because I am always true to my word.

I know I am a one and only;   *Ostrich*
Even alone – I am never lonely.

I have the horse-power to keep going;   *Horse*
I will go with the way my life is flowing.

I can quiet my mind like the bats do;   *Bat*
I trust my instincts and follow things thru.

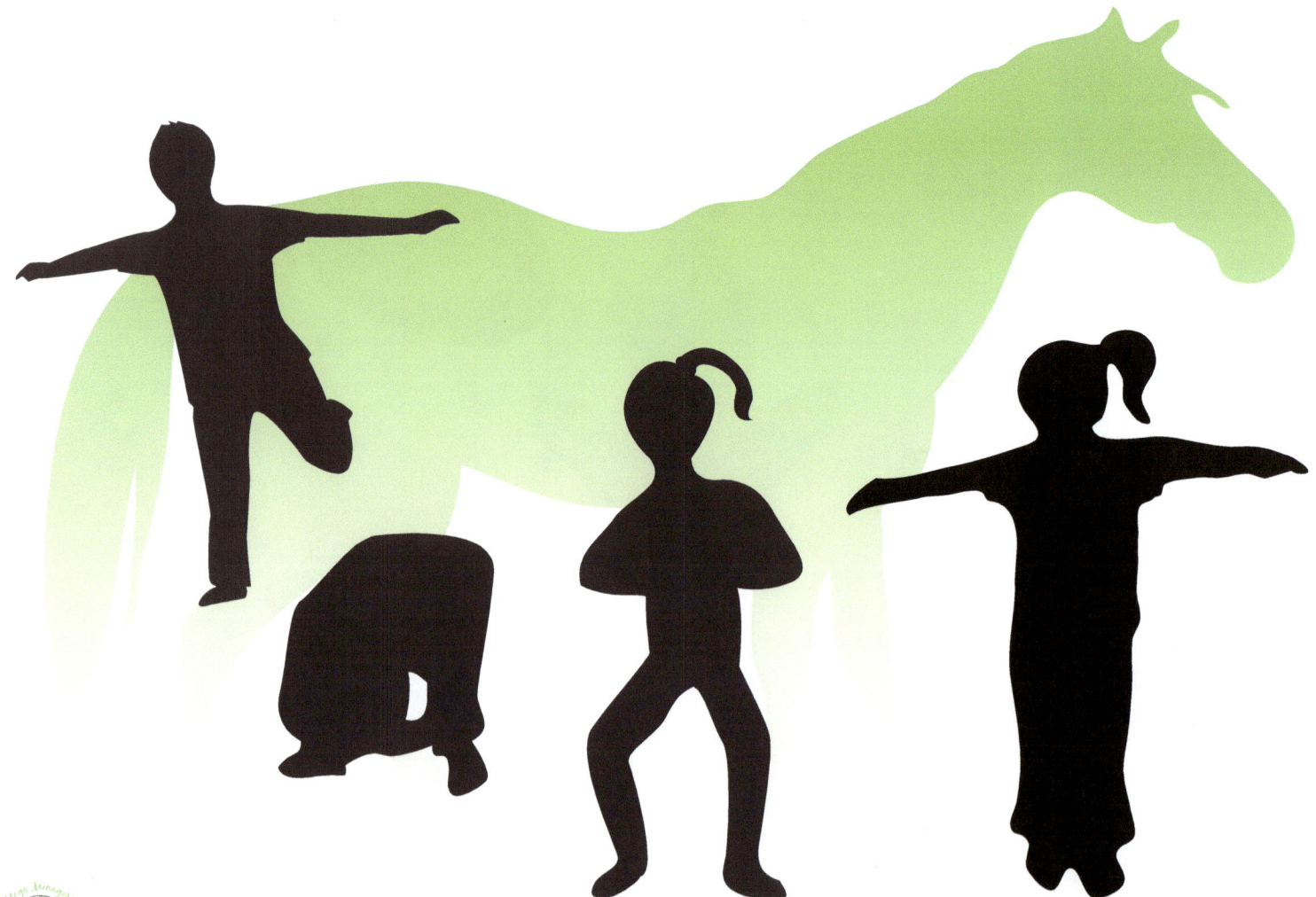

POSITIVE AFFIRMATION 17

I will persist thru the ups and downs;	*Frog*
All of my obstacles I hop around.	
I can unravel problems that I've found;	*Spider*
Like a spider I angle around.	
I am determined like a butterfly;	*Butterfly*
I won't let my dreams go passing me by.	
Like an owl I live in the moment;	*Owl - Right*
I can observe without passing judgment.	*Owl - Left*

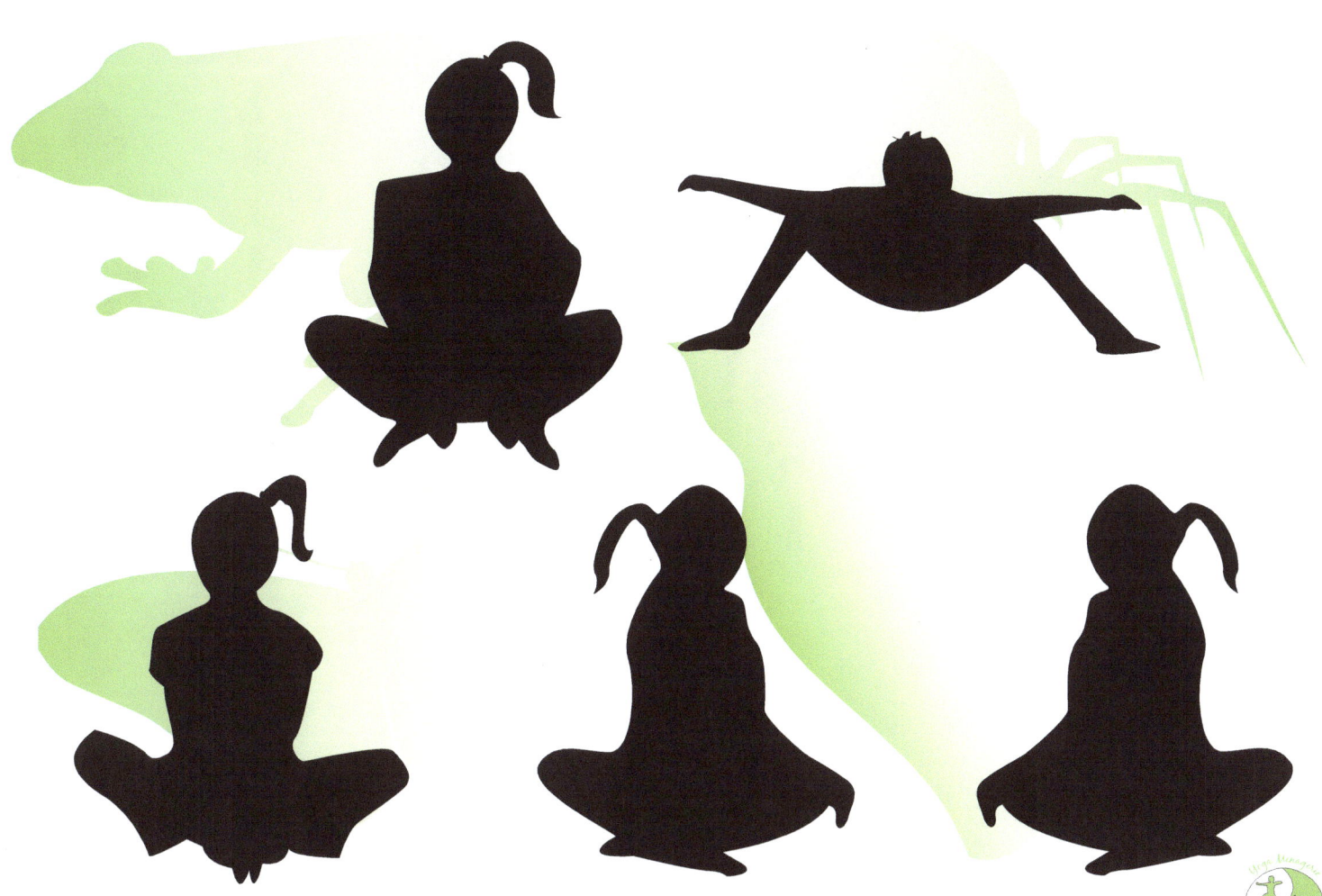

POSITIVE AFFIRMATION *18*

I am always seeking clarity; I spread out my limbs just like a tree.	*Tree*
Sometimes I'm a bird flying free; Sometimes I'm a flamingo and want to just be.	*Bird* *Flamingo*
I know I can accomplish anything; It is my true self that I'm claiming.	*Warrior 1 – Right* *Mountain/Palm Press*
I know my life is a blessing; Because my path is of my choosing.	*Warrior 1 – Left* *Mountain/Palm Press*

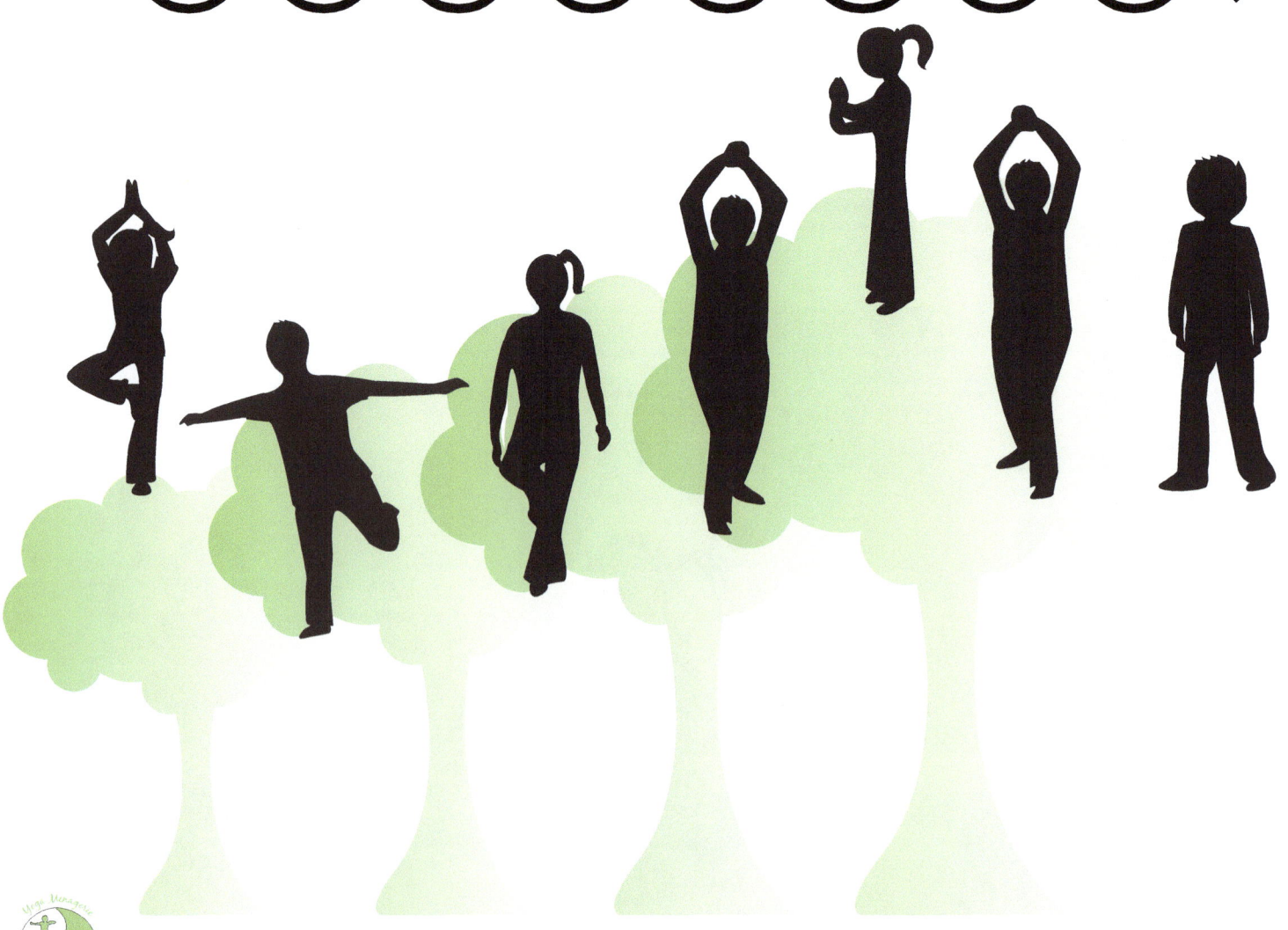

Yoga Journaling 1

Journal your answer or list 3 -5 descriptive words for each question-before and after you perform The Positive Affirmation Flows.

HOW AM I FEELING PHYSICALLY? WHAT AM I FEELING IN MY BODY? _____

_____

_____

HOW AM I FEELING MENTALLY? WHAT EMOTIONS AM I FEELING? _____

_____

_____

HOW DO I FEEL ABOUT MY LIFE? _____

_____

_____

After you have performed "The Positive Affirmation Flows" please answer the following questions.

WHAT CHANGES DO YOU NOTICE IN YOURSELF (MENTALLY, PHYSICALLY, IN YOUR LIFE)? ___

_____

_____

WHAT IMPROVEMENTS/CHANGES WOULD YOU LIKE TO HAVE IN YOURSELF AND YOUR LIFE? _____

_____

WHAT CAN I DO TO BE MORE POSITIVE PHYSICALLY AND MENTALLY? _____

_____

WHAT CAN I DO TO BRING MORE POSITIVITY TO MY LIFE AND THOSE AROUND ME? _____

_____

_____

POSITIVE AFFIRMATION RE'FLEX'IONS

Chapter Two

POSITIVE AFFIRMATION 1

I respect myself and I respect you;
I honor our relationship too.

Mountain/Palm Press-Palm Press–Up
Open hands /Reach up ---Clasp Hands

I am here, and want to be with you;
Together we see all things thru.

Warrior 2
Reach Over – Clasp Hands

I am connected to you as you are
to me;
And we are connected to all things
that be.

Lunge Forward

Feet Together –Stand up – Arch back

I will be there for you;
I will support you too.

Chair
Lean Back and Forward

I can open up and speak my mind;
Our hearts and our thoughts are
completely aligned.

Tree
Arms Up then Out to Side

POSITIVE AFFIRMATION 2

I care about you with all of my heart;
Everyday gives us a brand new start.

Star (Back to Back/Palms touching)
Raise hands up and to the side

I do my best to cooperate with you;
I do my best to be flexible too.

Twist Right
Twist Left

I am always honest when I talk to you;
I choose my words carefully and always
speak true.

Forward/Backward Bends
(Partners in Opposition)

I am always willing to help if you ask;
Together we can perform any task.

Triangle – Right
Triangle - Left
(Partners in Opposition)

POSITIVE AFFIRMATION 3

I am listening when you speak;
I recognize your thoughts are unique.

(Partners in Opposition)
Owl Twists
(Right/Left – Facing each other)

I care about the way you are feeling;
I share your emotions and want to aid in your healing.

Boat (1/2 and full)

I am here for you; we are present in the now;
I always will be, and this I vow.

Bear – Forward and Back
Reverse

I enjoy sharing my life with you;
And I appreciate the things you do.

Arms up – grab just right hands
Lean back and to the side

I trust in you to do what is right;
I believe in you and your insight.

Reach up and repeat in reverse

To my heart I am always true;
With all I am, I truly love you.

Lean forward – one person over the other

POSITIVE AFFIRMATION 4

I am proud that our relationship is strong;
With you is where I belong.

Butterfly (Lean forward / backward)
(Partners in Opposition)

Our relationship continues to grow;
We follow the rhythm of our own tempo.

Mermaid Twists – Clasp hands
Swoop around to lying back – and
swoop back around to mermaid
(Partners in Opposition)

I am happy with us and feel fulfilled;
Our future together is ours to build.

Reverse

I know I can always lean on you;
There is nothing we can't do!

Lace elbows and stand up together

POSITIVE AFFIRMATION RE'FLEX'IONS

Chapter Three

1

I love to share this time with you; Look at all the things that we can do.	*Mountain (hold hands)* *Turn head (R,L,Circle)*
When we work with each other we really shine; Because when we're together; we'll always be fine.	*Star* *Twists (R, L)*
No matter what happens to you or to me; There is no place I'd rather be.	*Triangle - R* *Triangle - L*
I'll always be there thru the ups and the downs; You can always count on me to be around.	*Chair* *Mountain*

2

Two little birds sitting in a tree; Looking at the clouds, happy as can be.	*Bird/Tree* *Hands up/Mt*
Two Little Birds stretch their wings so high; Then two little birds take off into the sky.	*Arms to side* *Bird*

3

No matter how near; No matter how far; I will always be there; No matter where you are.	*Mt /Warrior 2* *Reach over grasp hand*
You can always lean on me; I'll hold you and you hold me.	*Forward Lunge* *Mountain*
Even when we're far apart; You are always in my heart.	*Warrior 2* *Reach over grab hands*
There's no place I'd rather be; Then somewhere it's just you and me.	*Forward Lunge* *Mountain*

4

Butterfly sit and play with me; We'll soar and play happy as can be.	*Double Butterfly* *Back and Forth Tilts*
Swoop down low then way up high; See the spider crawling by.	*Back and Forth Tilts* *Spider*
Spinning the web all around; Way up high and down on the ground.	*Reach Right* *Reach Left*
Look there's a great big bear; Sitting there without a care.	*Bear* *Reach Right*
Stretching out really deep; Then lying down to go to sleep.	*Reach Left* *Both Lay Forward*

5

We are shooting stars; Watch us take off and really go far.	*Double Star* *Lift up*
Together we can twist around; Over any obstacles that we've found.	*Twist – right* *Twist – left*
Sometimes we're low and sometimes we're high; No matter what happens – We'll always get by.	*Bend Forward/ Reach Up* *Arch Back*
We are amazing, special and bright; Together we fill the whole world with our light.	*Triangle – right* *Triangle – left*
You and I are an unstoppable crew; Let's make all our dreams come true.	*Double Star* *Lift Up*

Yoga Journaling 2

Journal your answer or list 3 -5 descriptive words for each question-before and after you perform The Positive Affirmation Flows.

WHICH POSE IS YOUR FAVORITE TO DO TOGETHER? WHY? _____
_____
_____

WHICH POSE IS THE EASIEST? WHICH POSE IS THE HARDEST? _____
_____
_____

**WHICH POSE OR FLOW IS THE MOST FUN TO DO? WHICH MAKES YOU FEEL
HAPPIEST?** _____
_____
_____

WHICH POSE MAKES YOU FEEL MOST SUPPORTED? _____
_____
_____

WHICH POSE BRINGS THE STRONGEST FEELINGS OF TOGETHERNESS? _____
_____
_____

WHAT IS YOUR FAVORITE THING TO SAY TO YOUR PARTNER? _____
_____
_____

WHAT IS YOUR FAVORITE THING TO HEAR FROM YOUR PARTNER? _____
_____
_____

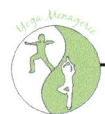

POSITIVE AFFIRMATION RE'FLEX'IONS

Chapter Four

Character Building Yoga
INSPIRED BY THE YAMAS AND NIYAMAS

The sequences contained within this chapter are designed to help mold and develop character. They promote strength, flexibility and balance both physically and mentally.

The concepts discussed in this chapter refer to universal principles; that are social and ethical guidelines or ideas to help promote living positively.

The Yamas refer to social behaviors; referring to how you treat others and the world around you. They are sometimes referred to as the "Don'ts" (i.e. don't steal, don't lie etc.)

The Niyamas refer to inner disciple or self-observance.; referring to how we treat ourselves. They are sometimes referred to as the "Dos" (i.e. do be clean, do be content, etc.)

When practiced regularly these concepts support positive transformation within the mind and body.

THE YAMAS
1. Ahimsa - Nonviolence
2. Satya - Truthfulness
3. Asteya - Nonstealing
4. Brahmacharya - Nonexcess
5. Aparigraha - Nonpossessiveness

THE NIYAMAS
1. Saucha - Purity
2. Santosha - Contentment
3. Tapas – Self-Discipline
4. Svadhyaya – Self-Study
5. Ishvara Pranidhana - Surrender

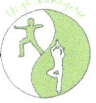

1 AHIMSA – NONVIOLENCE

Everyday I practice peace; I show compassion and kindness that doesn't cease.	*Noose - Right Mountain*
I never make judgments of things I don't know; I find out the answers and that way I grow.	*Noose - Left Mountain*
I let love guide my actions everyday; And I show to kindness in every way.	*Chair Mountain*
Harming none is truly key; That means anything or anyone- including me.	*Chair Mountain*

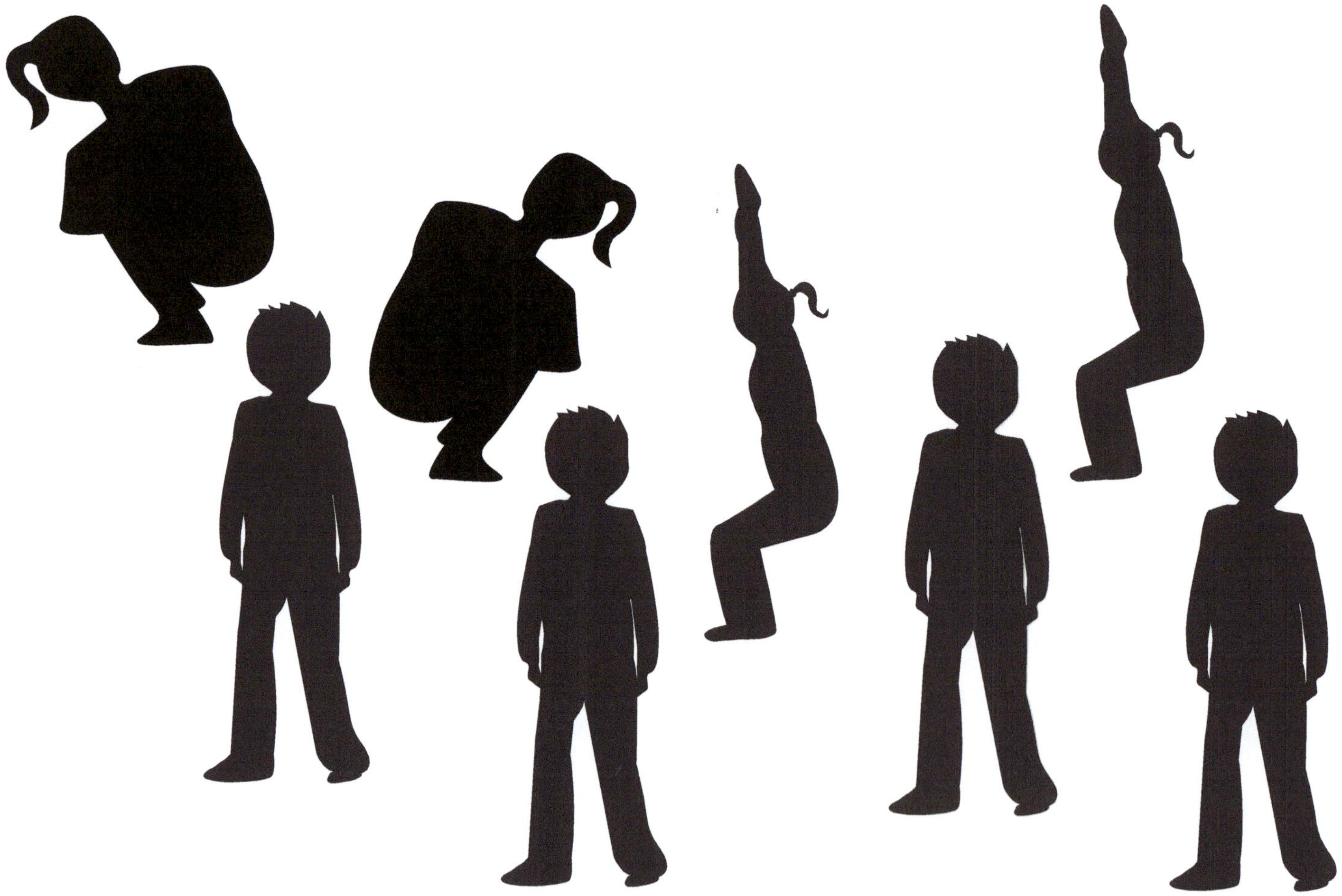

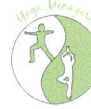

2 SATYA – TRUTHFULNESS

I let truthfulness guide me on my way;
I show sincerity in every way.

Warrior 1

I do not lie – My words are true;
I am genuine in all the things I do.

Flamingo
Horse

I am proud of my integrity;
I always behave respectfully.

Archer

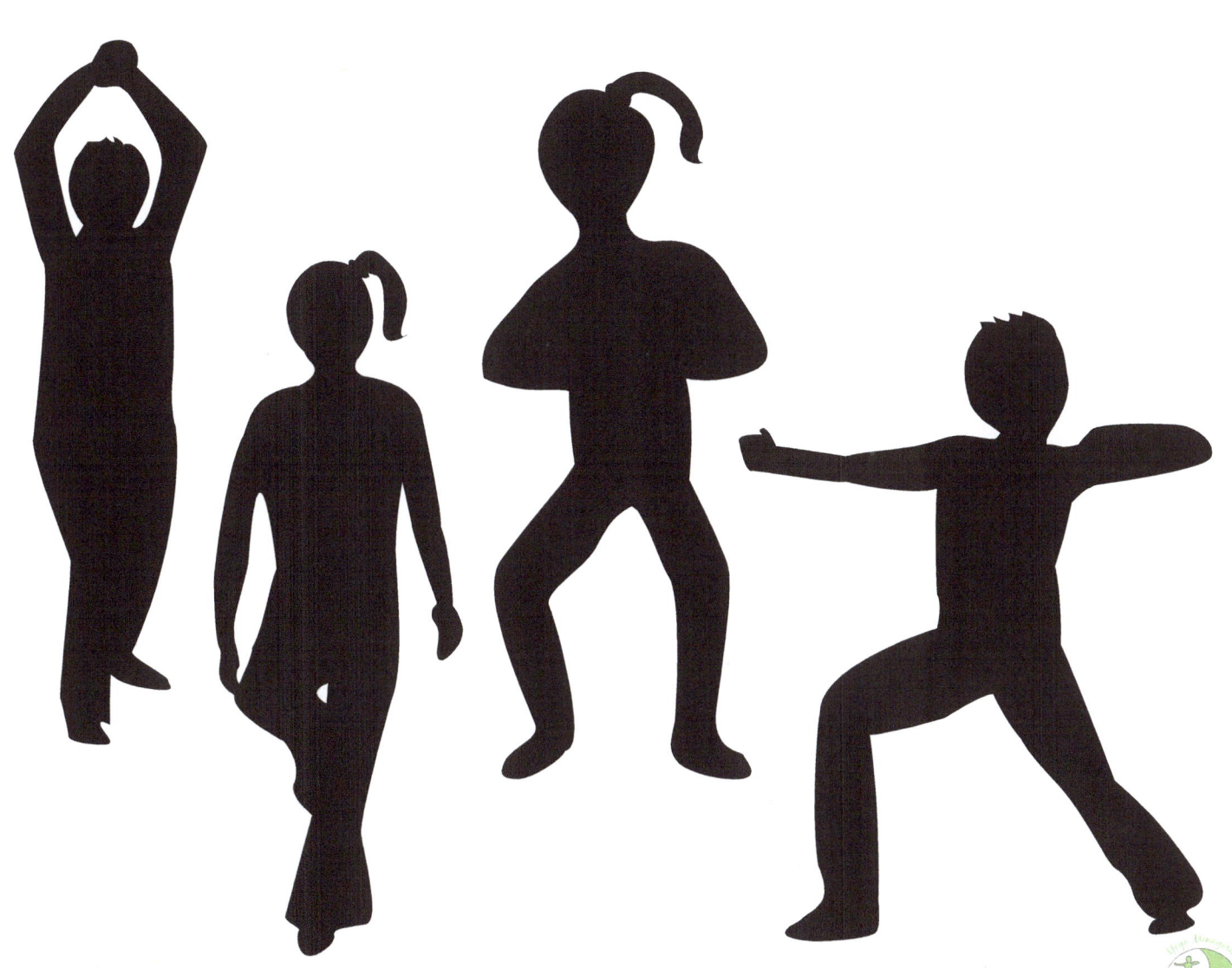

3 ASTEYA – NONSTEALING

I do not take – I do not steal;   *Gate – Left*
I always think of how others will feel.

I have abundance in everything;   *Camel*
And have no need to steal anything.   *Sunning Frog*

I only take things that are mine;   *Gate - Right*
I have all that I need and I am fine.

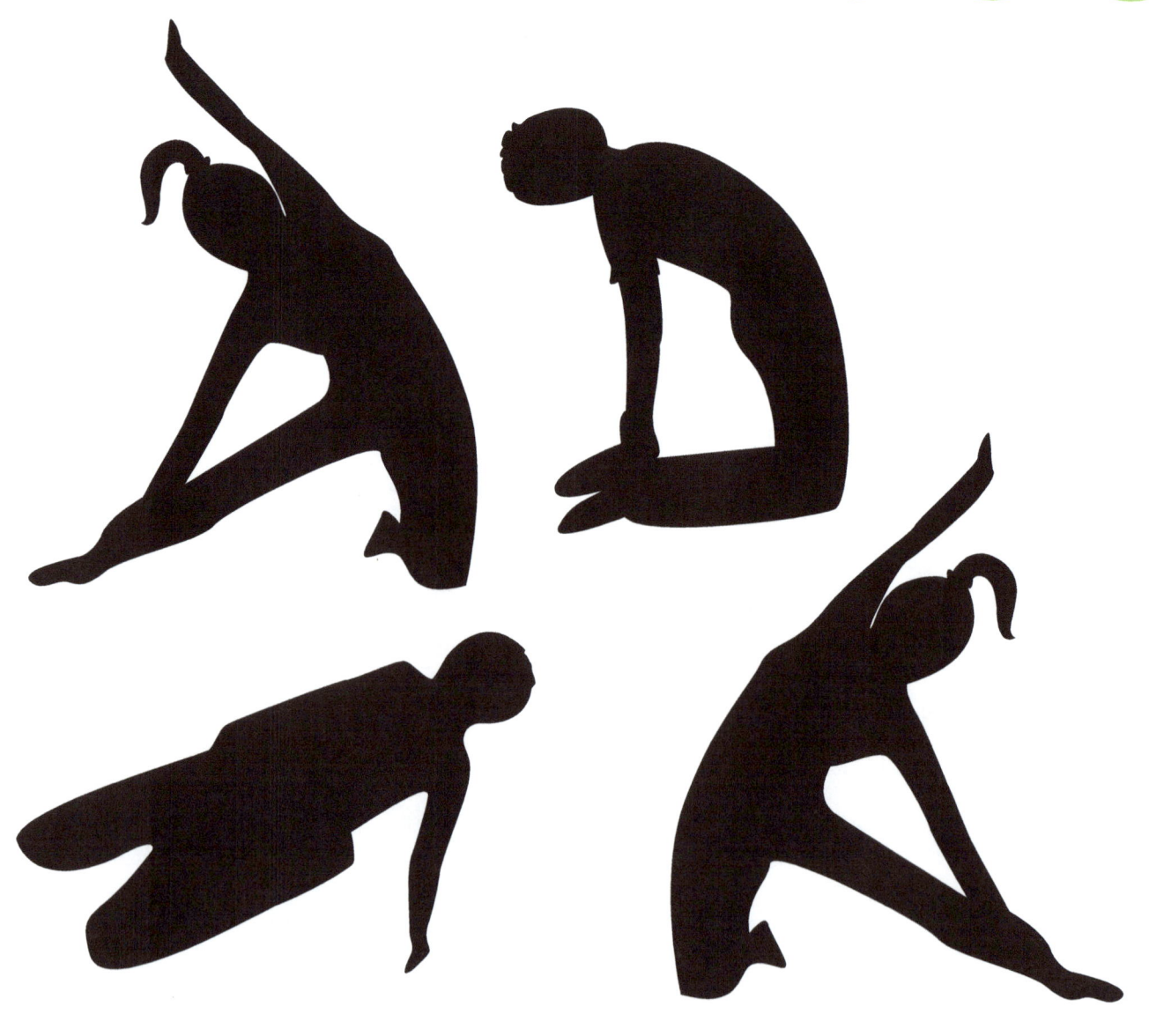

4 BRAHMACHARYA – NONEXCESS

I can have gains without excess;
And let others share in my success.

Lizard – Right
Plank

I use moderation in all of the things I do;
I keep my mind and body balanced too.

Lizard - Left
Peacock - Left

I am self-reliant and will follow my plan;
And along the way, I'll share all that I can.

Peacock - Right

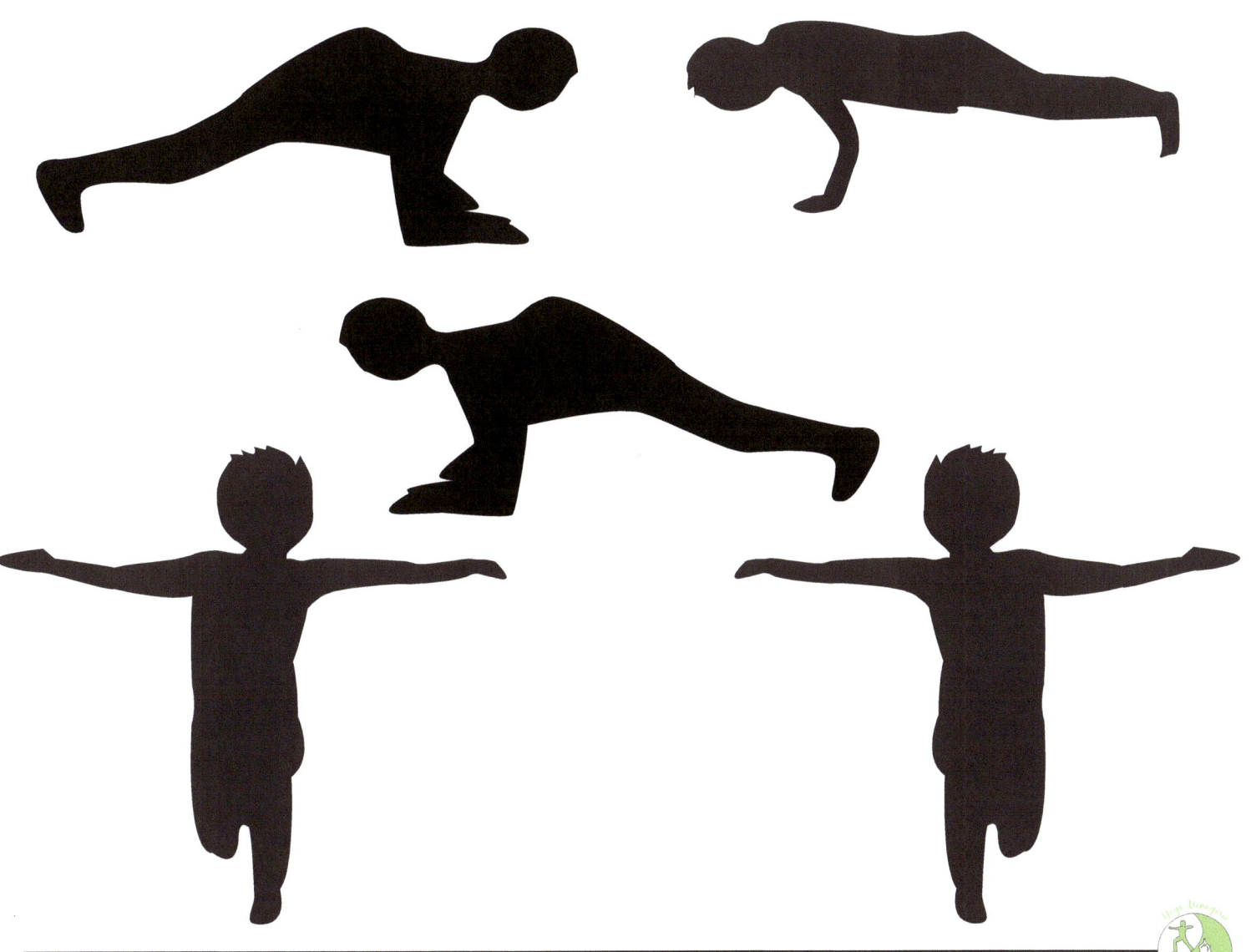

5 APARIGRAHA – NONPOSSESSIVENESS

I do my best to not be possessive; I don't hold onto things or act obsessive.	*Eagle – Right* *Star*
I let go of the things that I've outgrown; Moving past the negative things that I have known.	*Triangle* *Mountain*
There's no need for fear; I am safe here.	*Eagle - Left* *Star*
I release the things that prevent me- From moving forward to who I should be.	*Waterfall* *Bird*

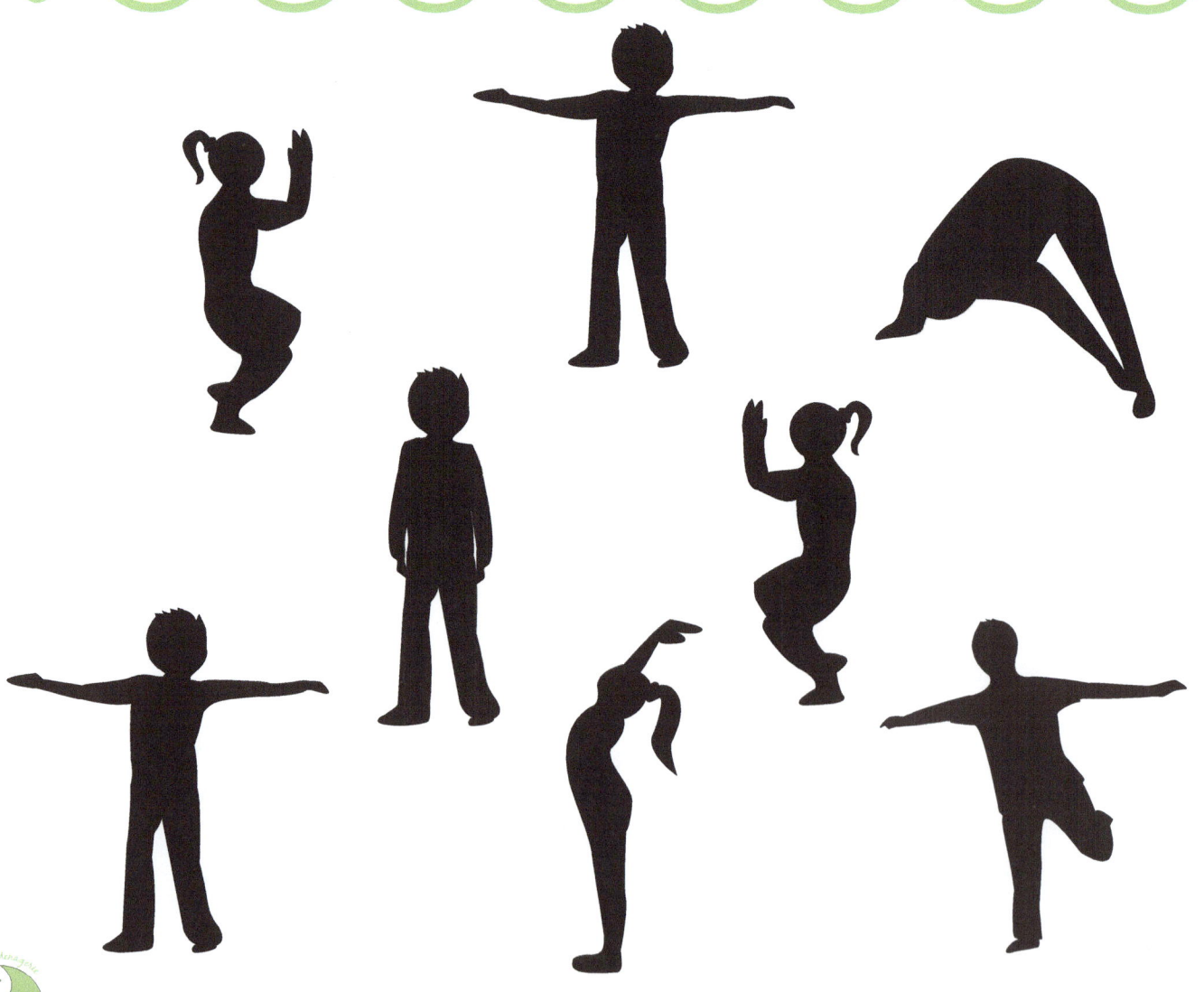

1 SAUCHA – PURITY

I take care of myself – inside and out;	*Cobra*
With cleanliness I am devout.	*Swan*
I keep my thoughts true and pure;	*Crocodile*
I keep my body clean for sure.	*Bow*
I pay attention to my mental needs;	*Crocodile*
And take great care with my physical deeds.	*Shark*
I treat myself with great respect;	*Crocodile*
I let my mind and body connect.	*Down Dog*

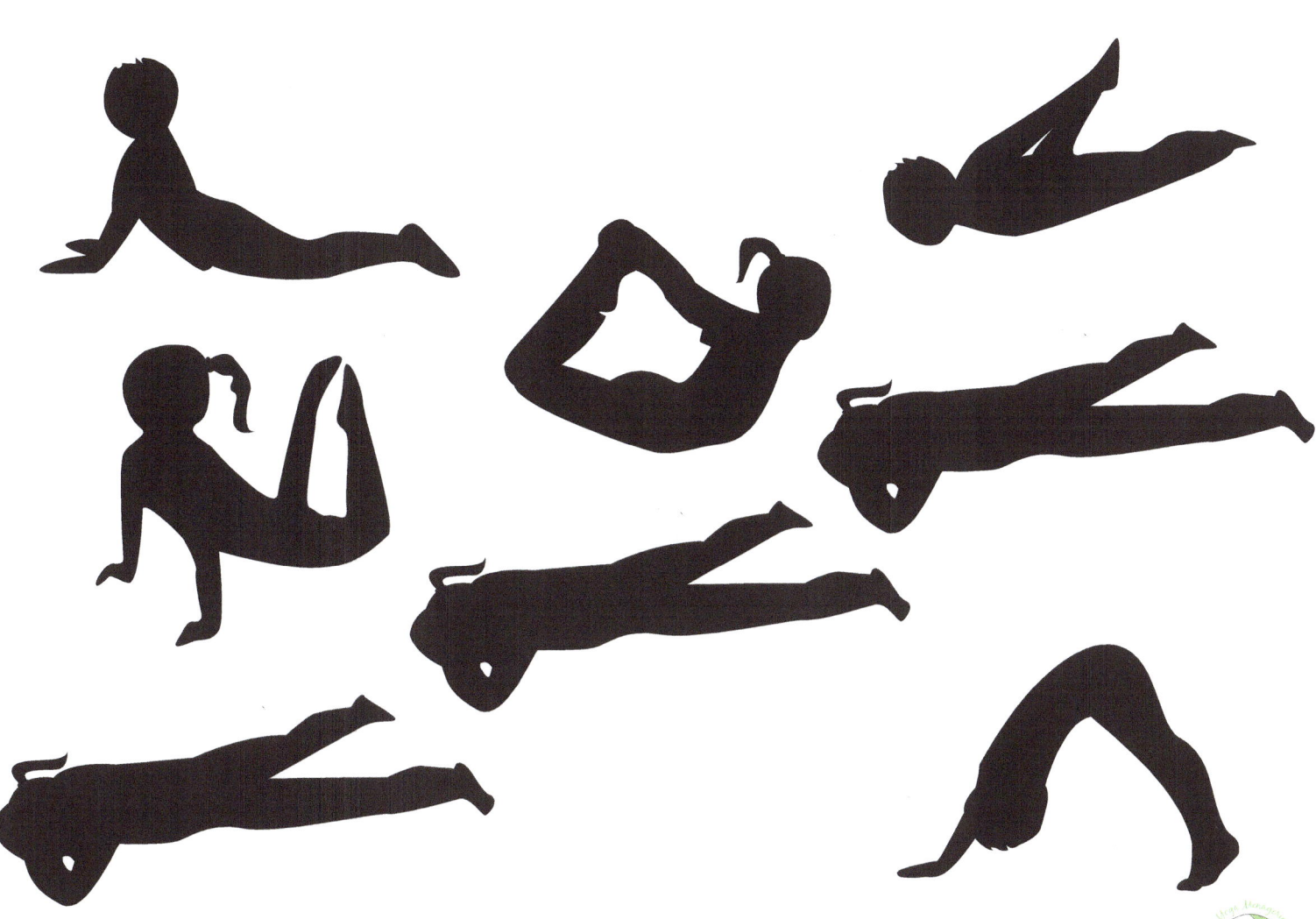

2 SANTOSHA – CONTENTMENT

I am at peace, I am content; I am at ease and can be present.	*Deer - Right* *Deer – Left / Staff*
I accept myself personally; And honor my individuality.	*Turtle*
I know I am a hidden gem; I 'm proud of who, what and where I am.	*Butterfly* *Flower*

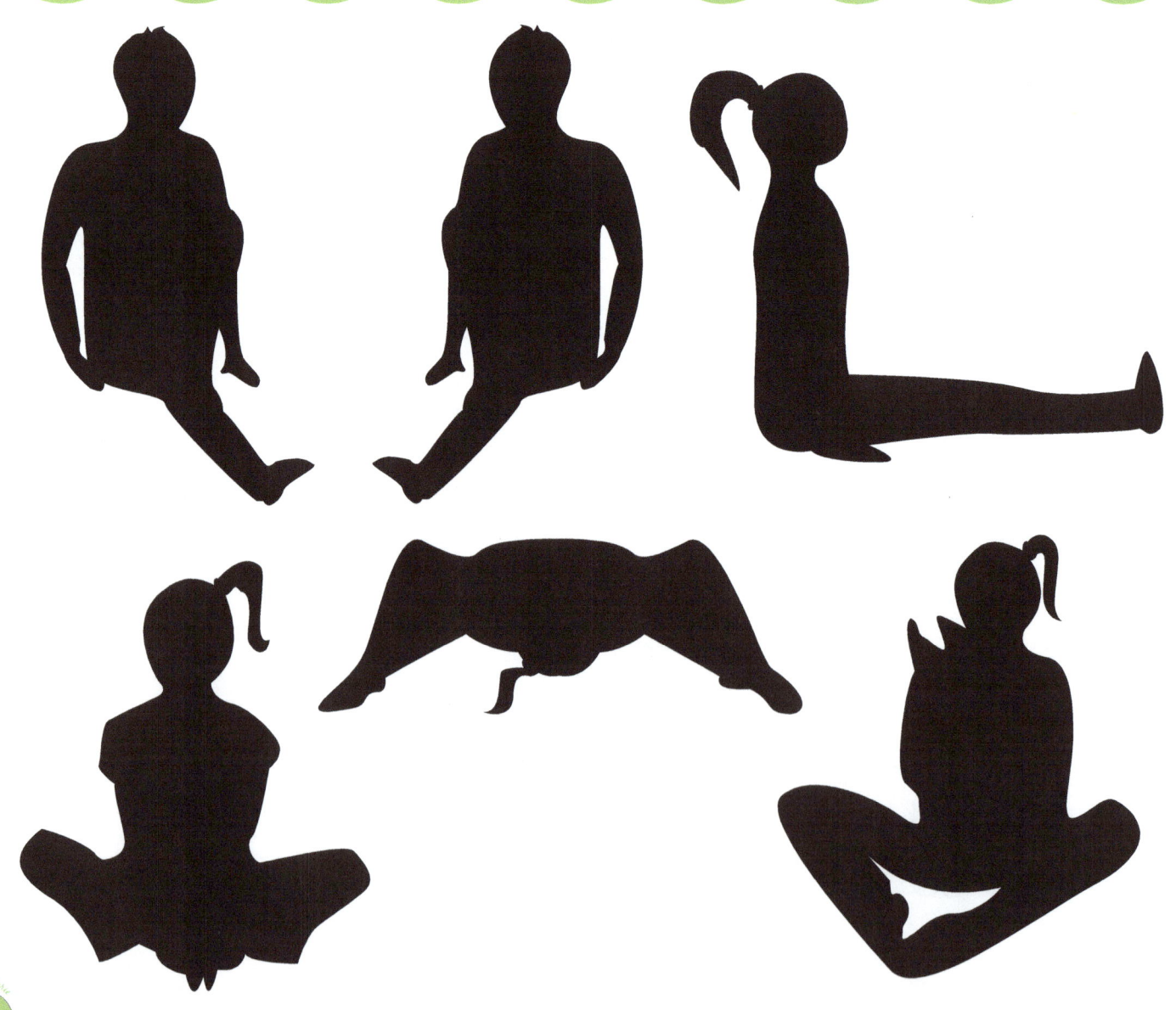

3 TAPAS – SELF-DISCIPLINE

I do my part – I do my share; I always pitch in because I care.	*Crescent Moon - Right* *Crescent Moon - Left*
I train my body and my mind; I work hard to keep them both aligned.	*Tree - Right* *Palm Press up*
I allow my awareness to expand and grow; I trust myself to go with the flow	*Volcano* *Triangle*
Self-discipline helps me to be at my best Gain control of my body and the thoughts I express.	*Tree - Left* *Star*

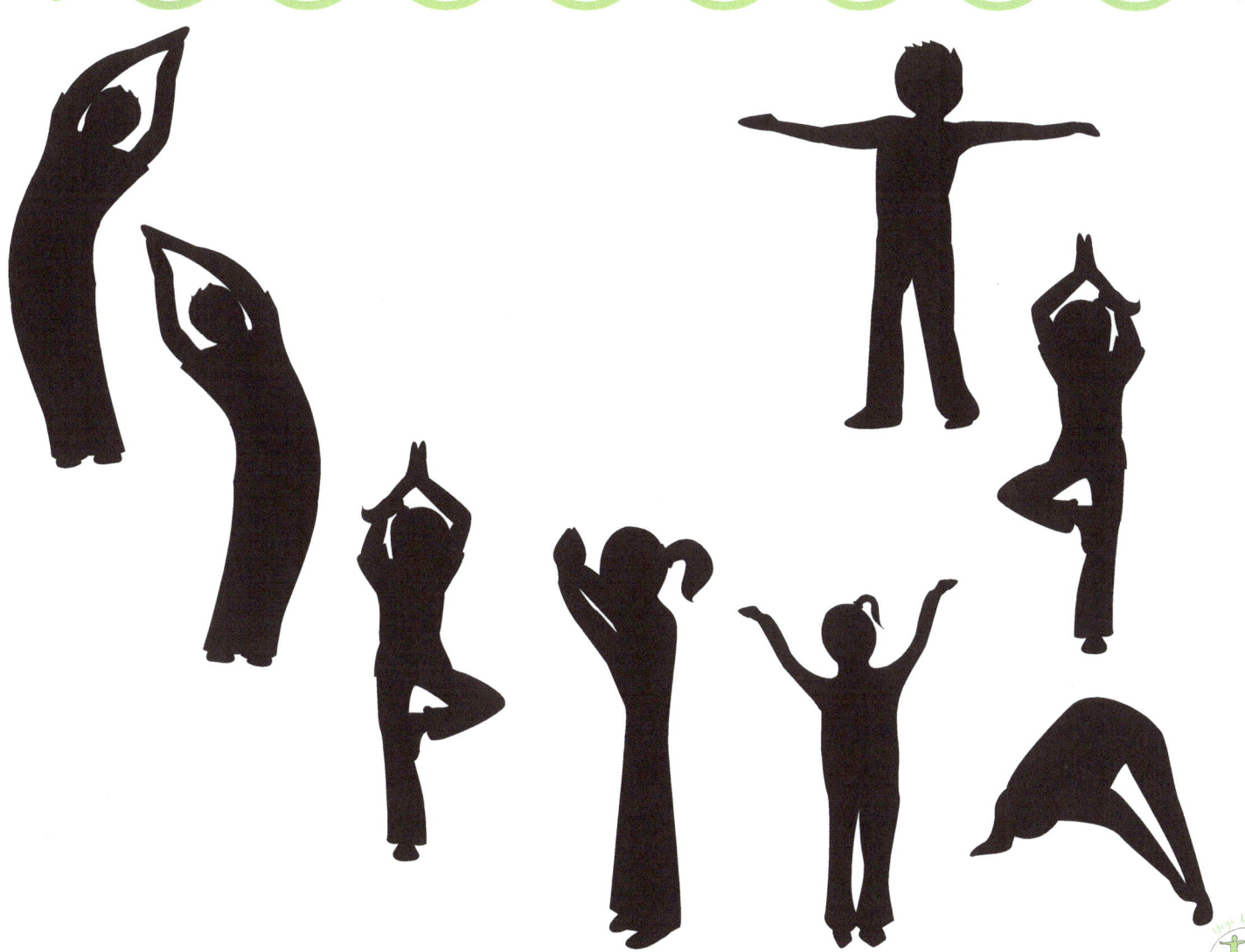

4 SVADHYAYA – SELF -STUDY

I take time to reflect upon me; What I am now and what I will be.	*Corpse* *Fish*
I recognize my own awareness; With myself I'm never careless.	*Bridge* *Crab*
I look inside to my inner core; Study myself down to every pore.	*Armadillo* *Candlestick*
I can find all the answers inside of me; I look within and set myself free.	*Table* *Plank - up*

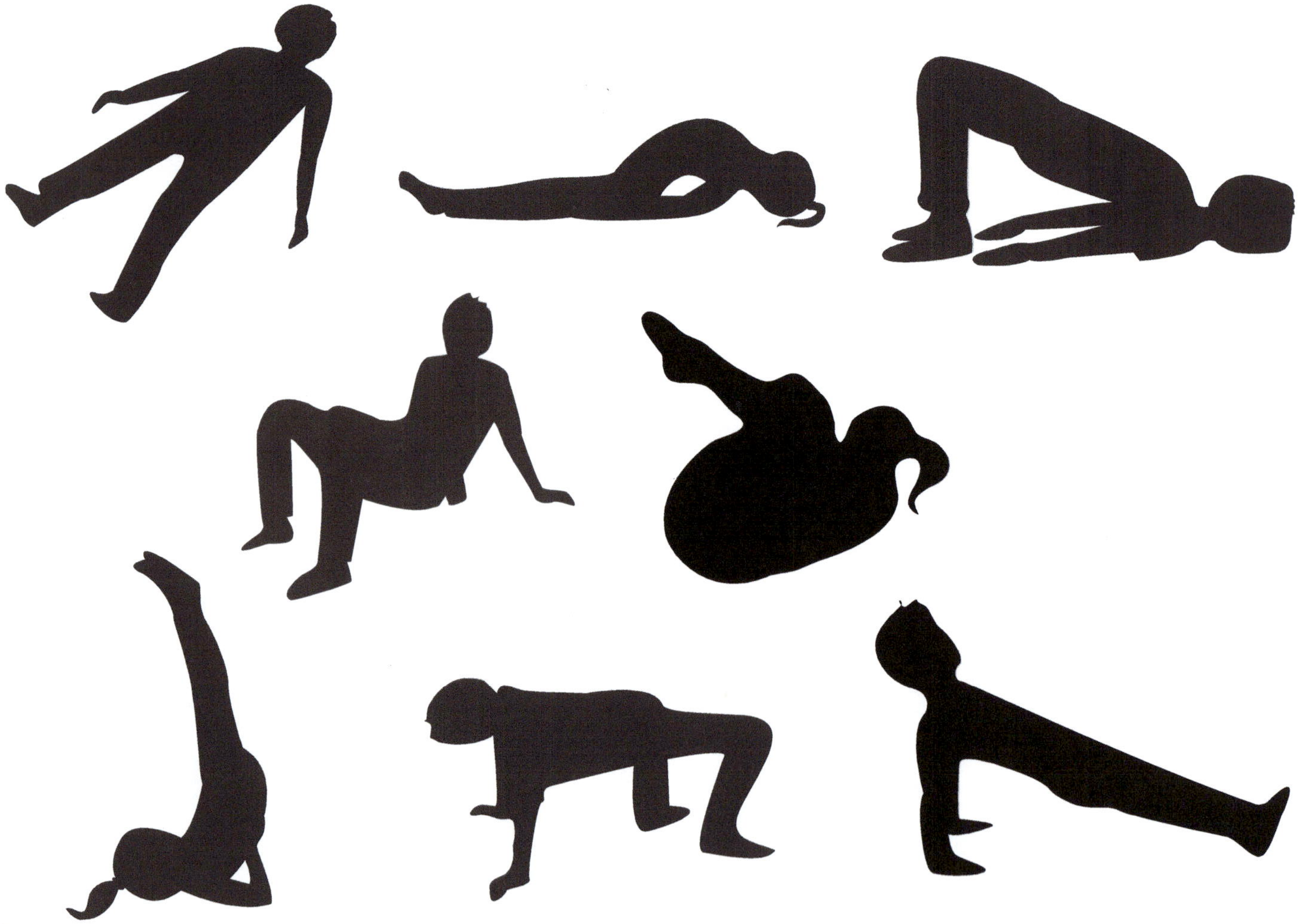

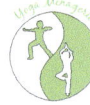

5 ISHVARA PRANIDHANA – SURRENDER

I trust the power inside of me	*Cat - Down*
I open my mind and set myself free.	*Cat - Up*
My awareness expands beyond what I see;	*Tiger – Right*
My consciousness grows into all it can be.	*Cat - Down*
I am mindful of what I say and do;	*Cat - Up*
I am humble in my thoughts and actions too.	*Tiger - Left*
I know in order to end all my strife.	*Cat - Down*
I must believe in myself and surrender to life.	*Sleeping Cat*

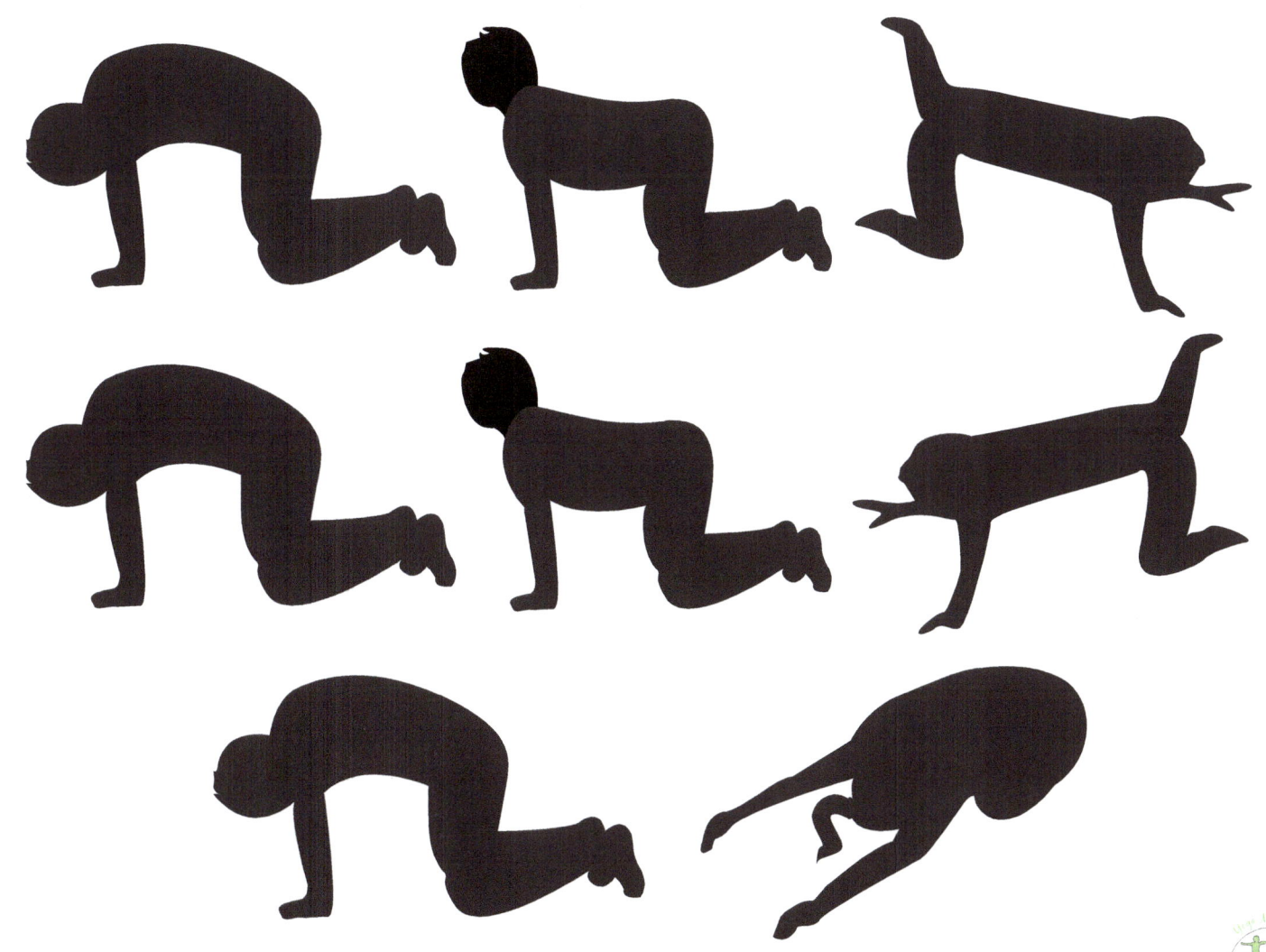

Yoga Journaling 3

The following questions can be used to journal for each sequence individually or for the entire Character Building section as a whole.

HOW DO YOU USE THIS CONCEPT IN YOUR DAILY LIFE? _____

_____

_____

WHAT DIFFICULTIES DO YOU FIND USING THE IDEA OR CONCEPT FROM THE SEQUENCE? HOW DO YOU OVERCOME THOSE CHALLENGES? _____

_____

_____

WHICH CONCEPT IS EASIEST TO UNDERSTAND? EASIEST TO PERFORM? _____

_____

_____

WHICH IS THE MOST DIFFICULT TO UNDERSTAND, USE OR PERFORM? _____

_____

_____

HOW DO THESE IDEAS RELATE TO YOUR OWN CORE VALUES? _____

_____

_____

HOW DO YOU SEE THIS CONCEPT IN THE WORLD AROUND YOU? WHICH CONCEPT WOULD YOU LIKE TO SEE MORE OF? WHY? HOW CAN YOU MAKE THIS HAPPEN?

_____

_____

_____

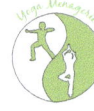

POSITIVE AFFIRMATION RE'FLEX'IONS

Glossary

Glossary

POSITIVE AFFIRMATION RE'FLEX'IONS (BOOK TWO)

ARCHER
Standing with feet apart - one foot facing front - the other facing the side; extend the same arm as foot facing to the side and use the other to pull back a bow (bent arm - pull hand to shoulder)

ARMADILLO
Sitting on the floor - curl body into a ball and rock backward and forward

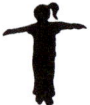
BAT
Stand feet together - arms extended out to the side - rise up on toes

BEAR
Sitting on the floor - extend legs out into a straddle and reach to the right, left and center

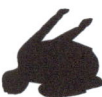
BEE
On knees- sit up and put arms behind you like wings then bring bend body forward to legs

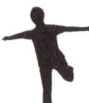
BIRD
Standing on one foot- lift the other leg behind you and bring your arms out to the side

BRIDGE
Lying on the floor - lift hips off the ground

BUTTERFLY
Sitting on the floor - bend legs and bring feet together

CAT TILTS UP
On the floor on hands and knees - arch back and look up

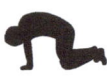
CAT TILTS DOWN
On knees - pull body back to sit on feet - arms extended and stretched out in front of you

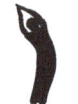
CRESCENT MOON
Standing feet together- hands clasped overhead- reach over to the side

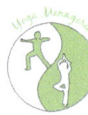

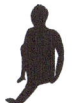
DEER
Sitting on the floor with legs extended in front of you - bend one leg into your chest and grab with your arms, then reverse

DOWN DOG
Place hands on the floor – feet apart- lift body into a "V" shape with the hips pointing up

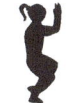
EAGLE
Cross one leg over the other and place arms to the side or behind you like wings and lean forward

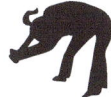
ELEPHANT
Standing feet spread apart - hands clasped together in front of you with arms extended out in front of you - bend forward then lift arms as trunk

FISH
Lying on your back on the floor - arch back off the floor

FLAMINGO
Standing on one leg – bend the other leg and place foot near knee or other foot

FLOWER
Sitting in butterfly - lift feet off ground or cup hands and lift up

FROG
Squat to floor and hop

GORILLA
Standing legs apart - bend forward and place hands or knees on floor

HORSE
Standing legs apart - knees bent - hands in prayer - arms bent with elbows out to the side

LION
Kneeling – scrunch hands and face and then extend arms forward and un-scrunch face - open mouth

MOUNTAIN
Standing straight up - arms down to your sides

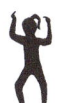
OPEN HERO
Standing legs apart – knees bent – arms extended out to the side and bent with hands pointing up

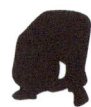
OSTRICH
Standing feet apart - cover head with arms and bend in half forward

OWL
Sitting on the floor- cross legs in front of you and reach one arm to the opposite side and twist then reverse

PEACOCK
Kneeling on one knee or lunge - extend arms behind you and lift up

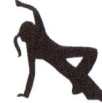
RAINBOW
On the floor facing the side - one leg straight with the other bent - lift hips off the ground - lift arm from side to your head and back down

ROCK - CHILD'S POSE
Kneeling on the floor lie chest on knees

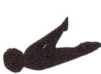
SHARK
Lying on the floor - clasp hands behind you and lift up to create a fin

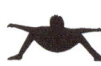
SPIDER
In squat or on the floor with legs bent - arms extended out the side

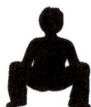
SQUAT
Legs bend with hands touching the floor

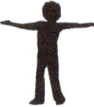
STAR
Standing feet apart with arms extended out to the side

SUN
Standing feet together - round arms over head

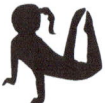
SWAN
On the floor lying on your stomach – lift feet up and roll head back

TREE
Standing on one leg - bend the other leg and bring the foot to touch the knee - hands in prayer

TRIANGLE
Standing feet apart – bend forward and touch your toes- right, left and center

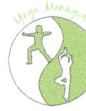

TURTLE

Sitting on the floor - legs bent out the side - place arms under your knees and hands behind feet then tuck head down

VOLCANO
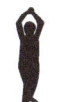
Standing in mountain pose - hands in prayer - lift hands over head then open them and bring arms down to your sides

WARRIOR 1
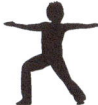
Standing with leg straight with foot facing the side – other leg placed in front slightly bent- clasp hands and raise overhead

WARRIOR 2
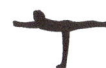
Standing with leg straight and foot facing the side- other leg placed in the front slightly bent - reach arms out to the side and then lift front arm up and arch body back

WARRIOR 3

Standing on one leg the other extended to the back – arms extended in fron2

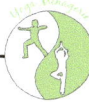

POSITIVE AFFIRMATION RE'FLEX'IONS

Re'flex'ion Cards

The Positive Affirmation Re'flex'ions cards
can be used in a variety of ways.
Each card contains a positive affirmation
and a corresponding yoga pose.
This is great way to engage children and teens
in exercise, reading out loud and meditation.
Use these cards daily for morning or evening re'flex'ions,
or when you need a yoga pick me up
at any time throughout the day.
These cards can be adapted for various uses
at home and in numerous ways
in the classroom!

ARCHER POSE

I am determined, I will never stop; like an archer, I always take my shot.

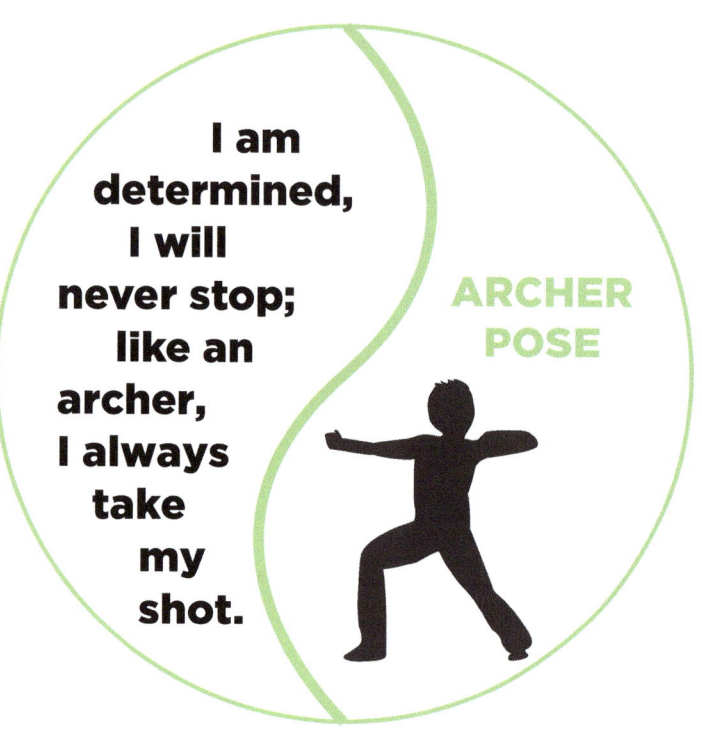

COBRA POSE

I am clever and cunning like a snake; I put great effort into everything I make.

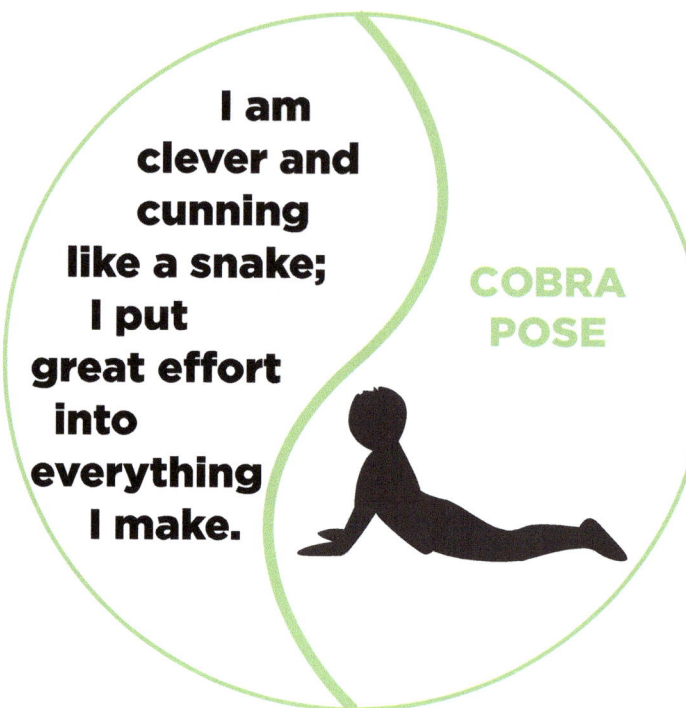

DOG POSE

I am honest, fair and true; just like a dog I'm loyal too.

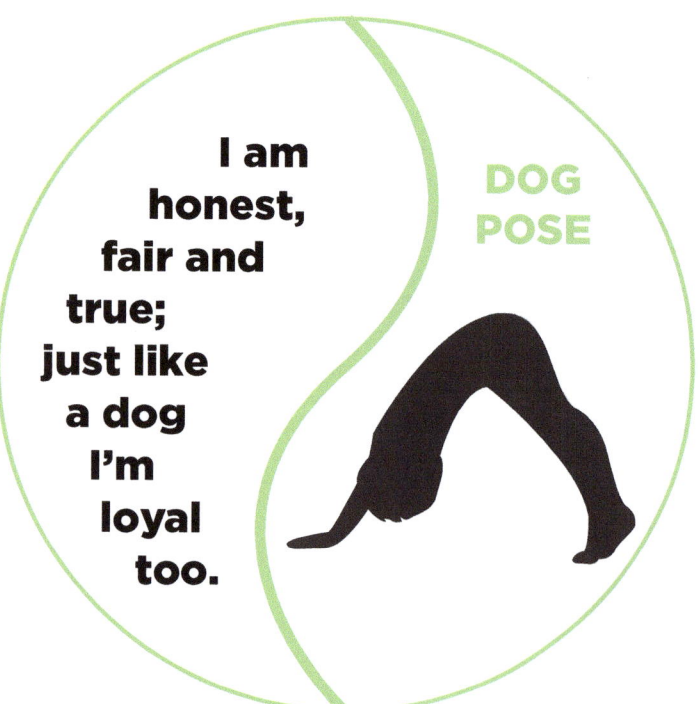

MOUNTAIN POSE

I am alert and aware of everything around me; I am content that all things are as they should be.

I am a rock, solid and strong, I know exactly where I belong.

ROCK POSE

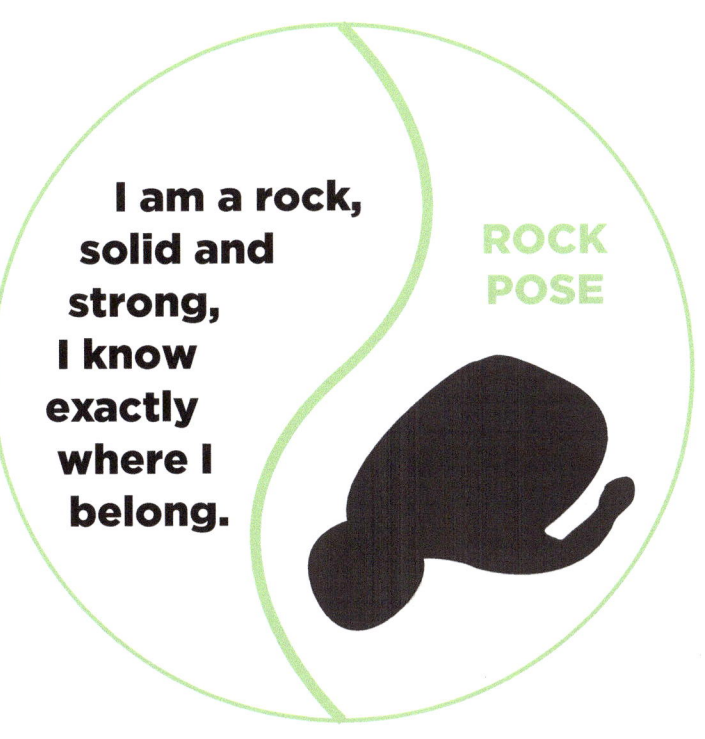

I sparkle like a twinkling star, I share my light with those near and far.

STAR POSE

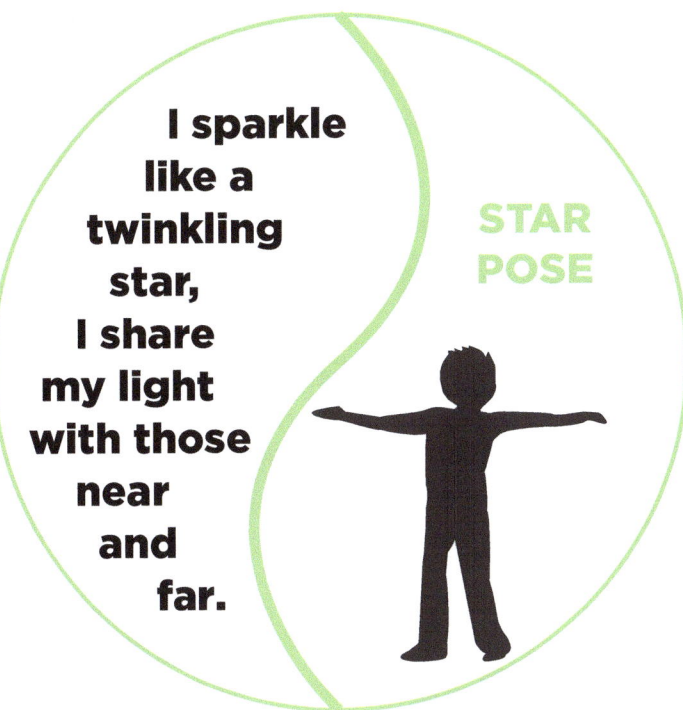

I open my heart so I can set free; all the love inside of me.

TABLE POSE

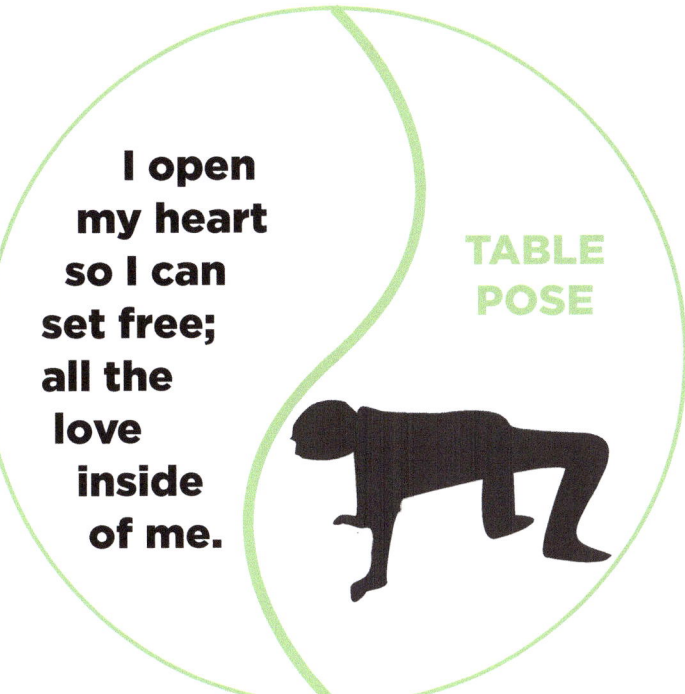

I can become anything if only I try, with my roots in the ground, I reach for the sky.

TREE POSE

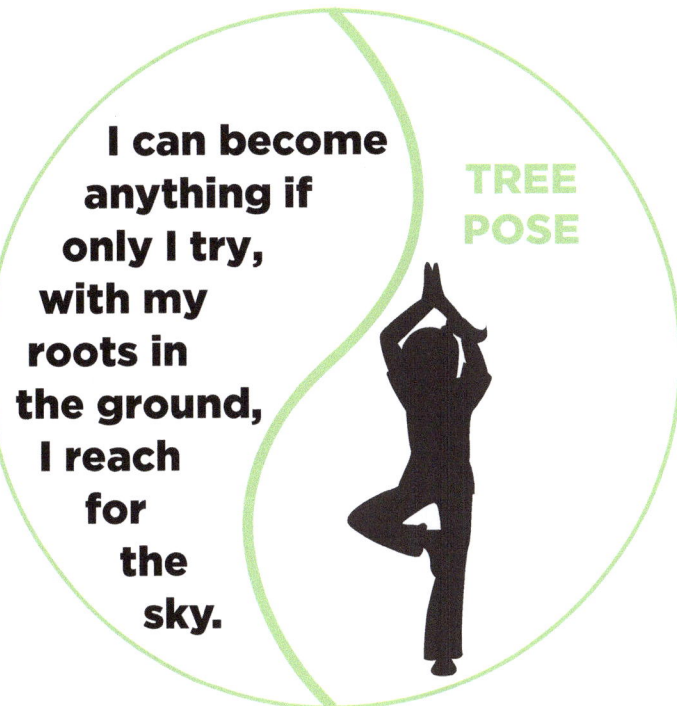

I am
as flexible
as a rainbow;
accepting
change
helps me
let go.

RAINBOW POSE

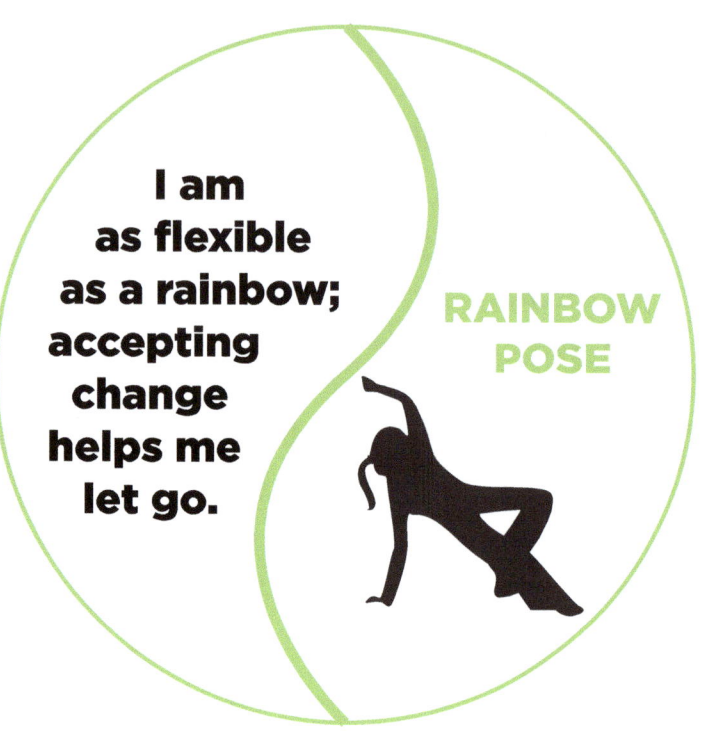

I can
surf on the
waves and
sail on the
tide;
whatever
I do I do
it with
pride.

WARRIOR 2 POSE

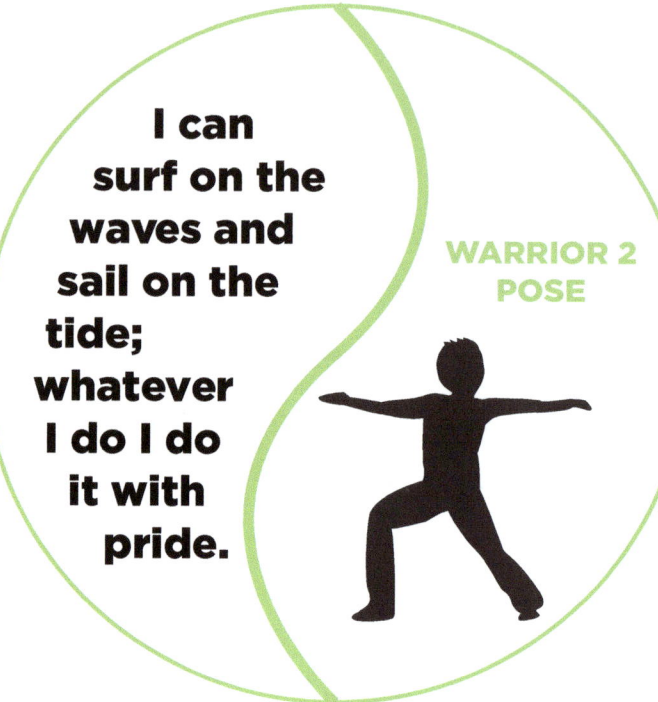

Like a
swan I'm
graceful
and sleek;
and I act
strong
when I
feel
weak.

SWAN POSE

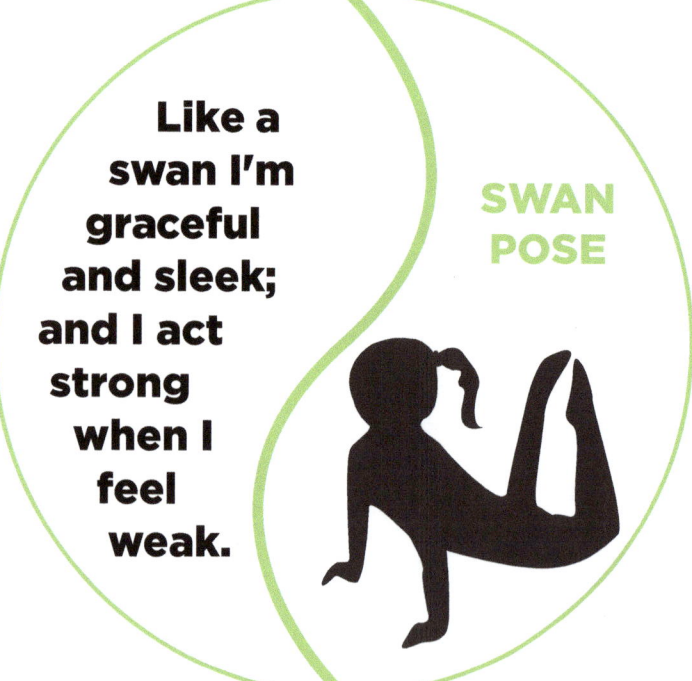

I am
bright and
vibrant like
the sun,
I shine
my light
on
every-
one.

SUN POSE

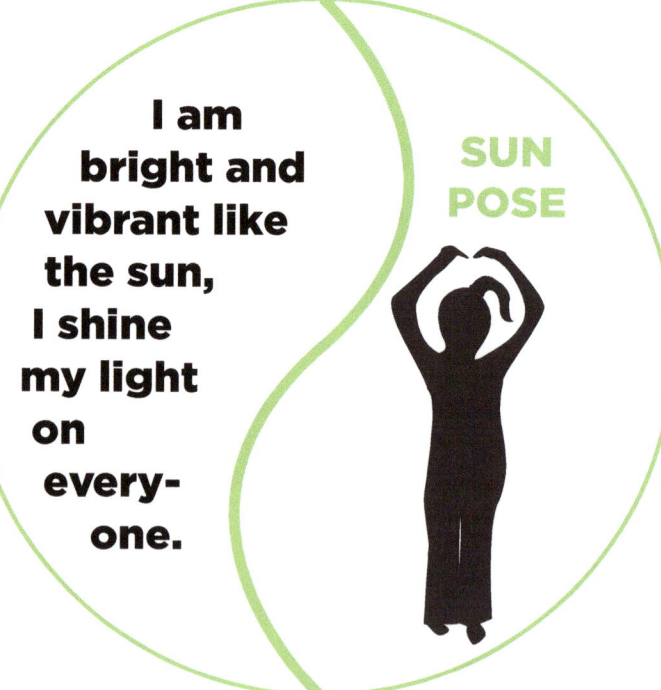

I am responsible like my friend turtle and I can carry myself over any hurdle.

TURTLE POSE

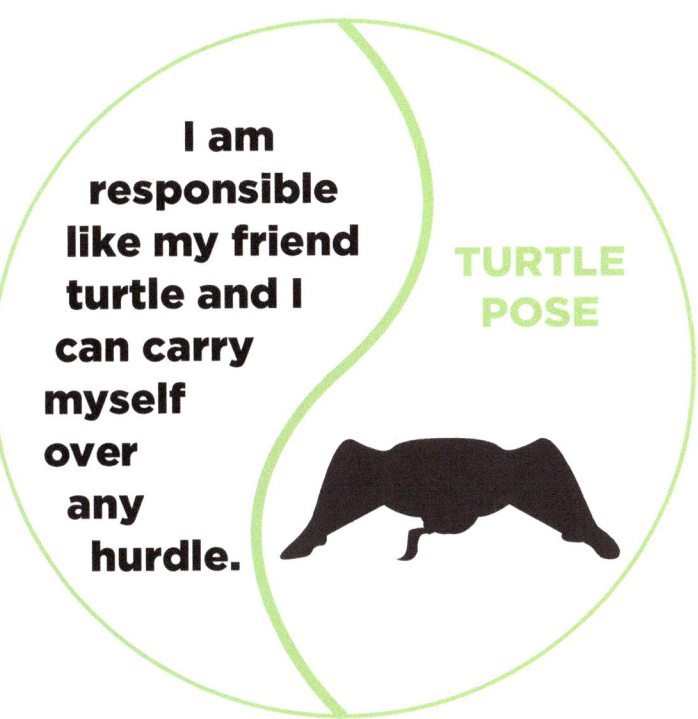

I keep on moving like a fish and I'll never stop till I get my wish.

FISH POSE

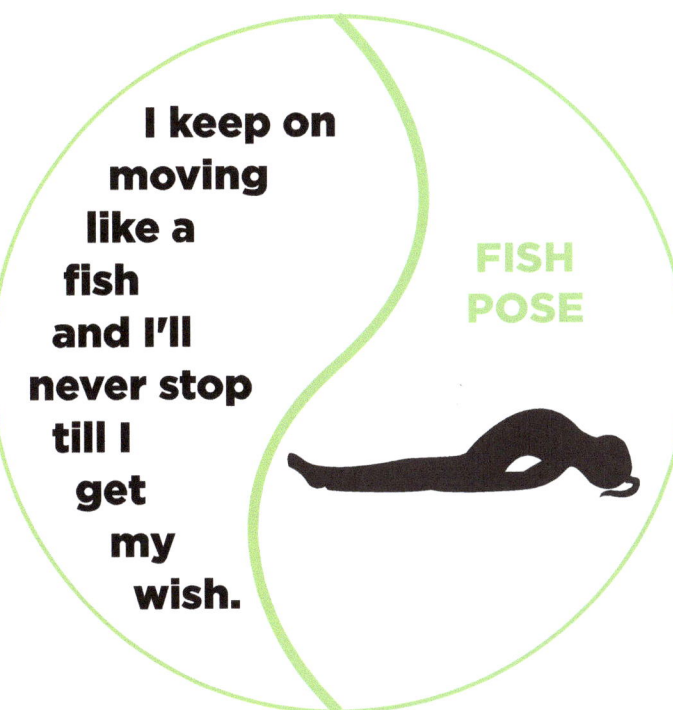

I am sure-footed like a flamingo; I trust myself and go with the flow.

FLAMINGO POSE

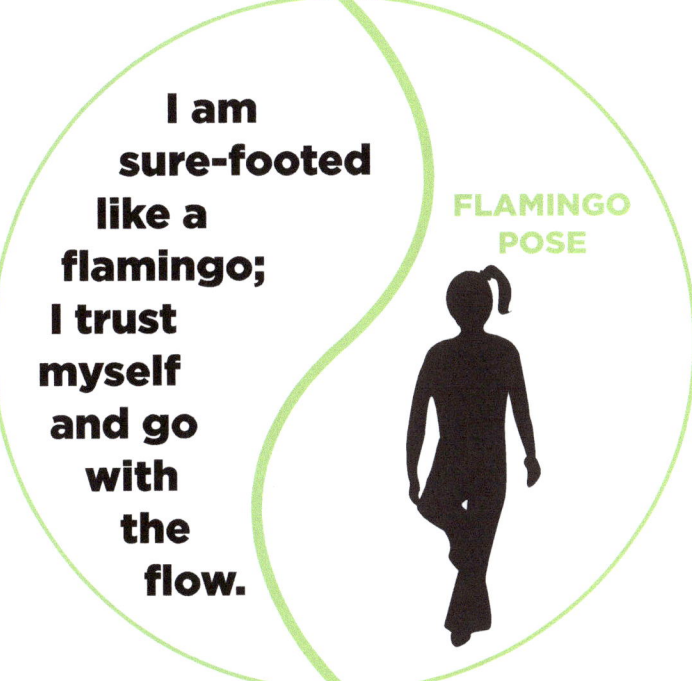

I am special like a tiny seed; watch me bloom and grow into me.

FLOWER POSE

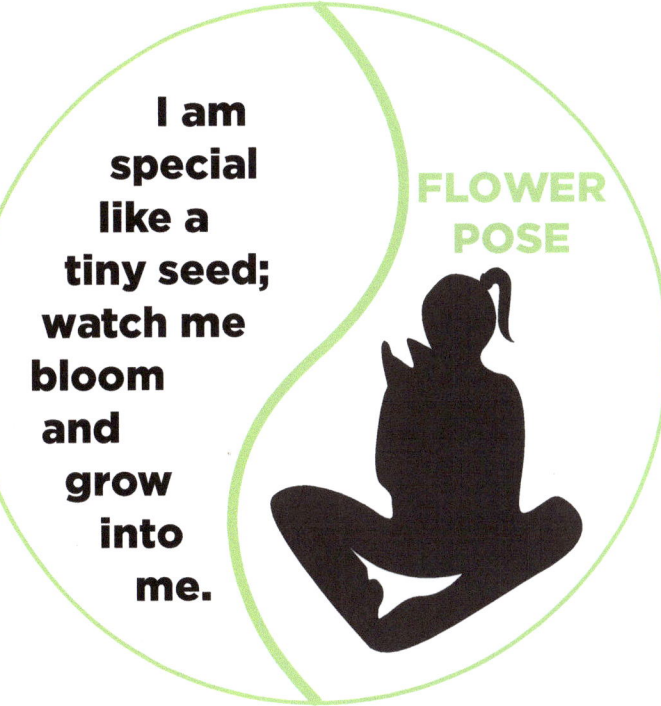

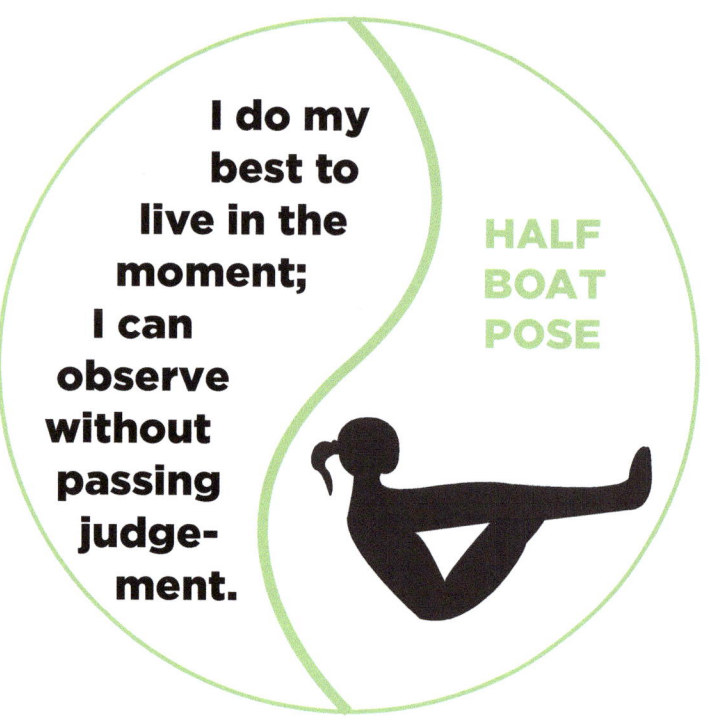

I do my best to live in the moment; I can observe without passing judge- ment.

HALF BOAT POSE

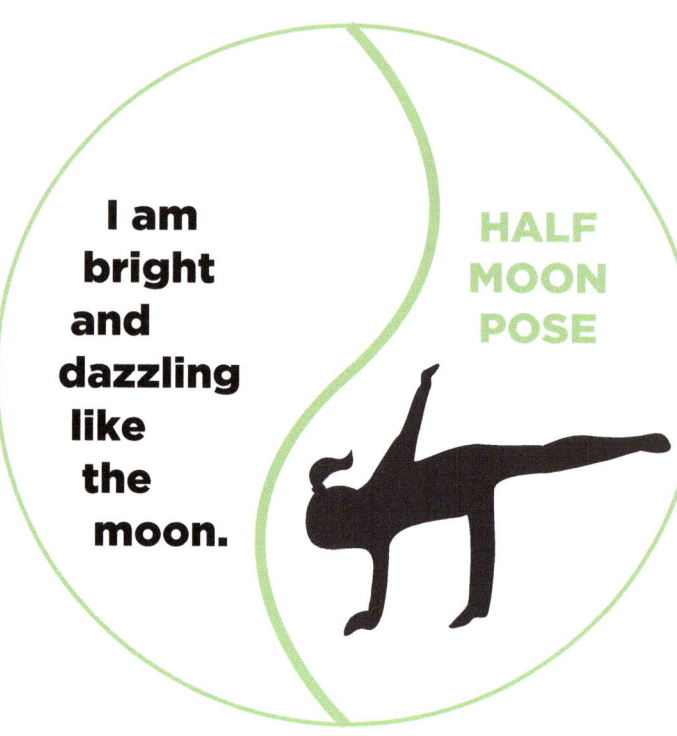

I am bright and dazzling like the moon.

HALF MOON POSE

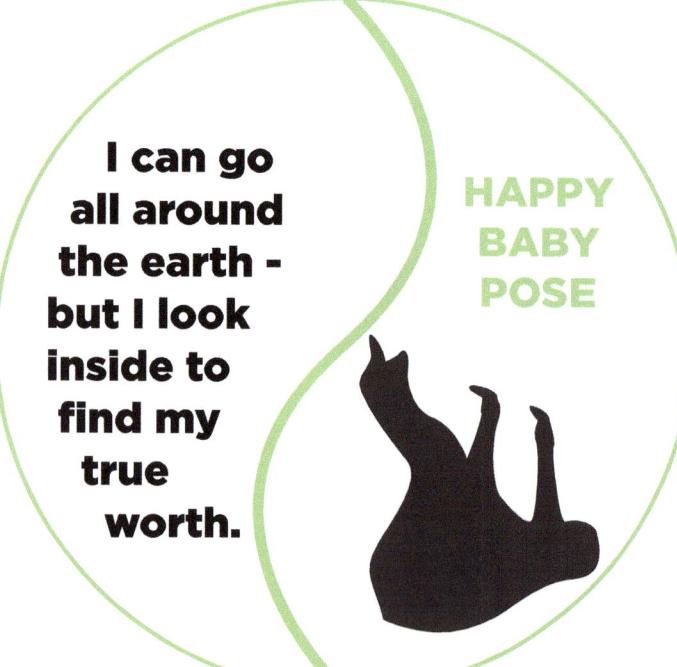

I can go all around the earth - but I look inside to find my true worth.

HAPPY BABY POSE

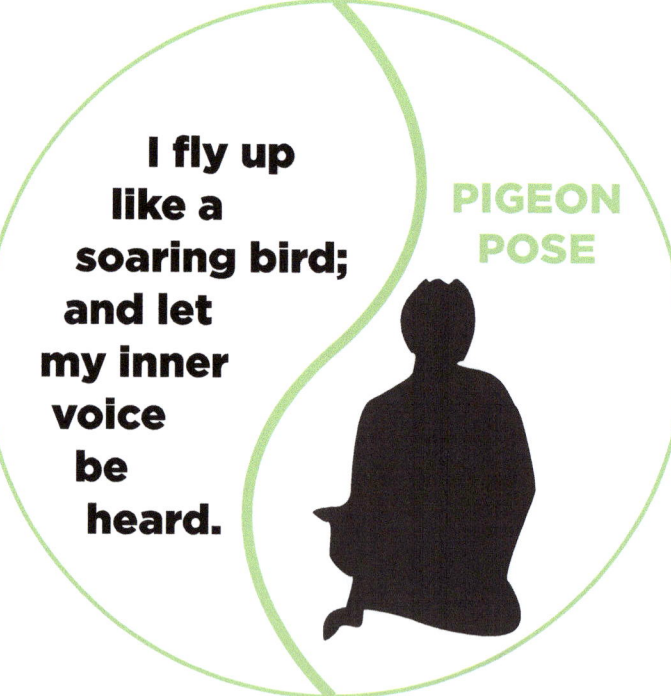

I fly up like a soaring bird; and let my inner voice be heard.

PIGEON POSE

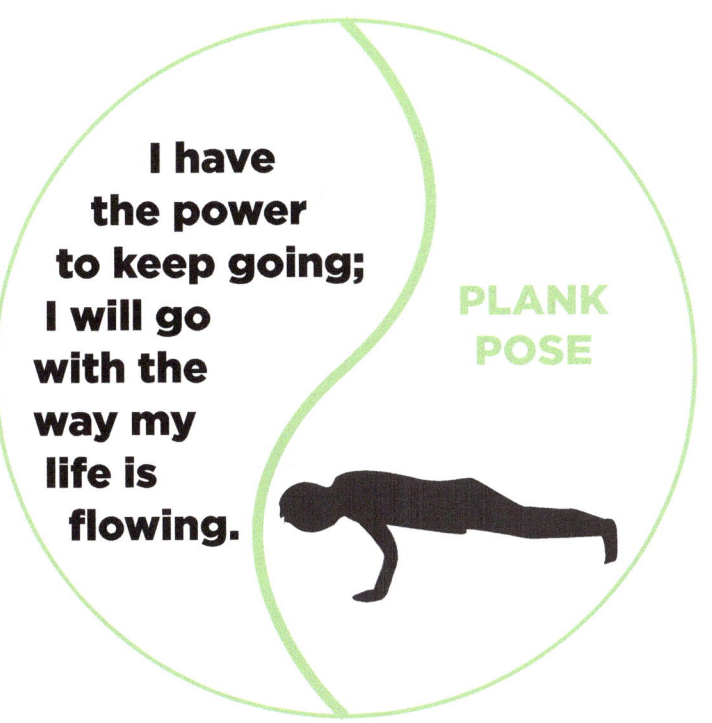

I have the power to keep going; I will go with the way my life is flowing.

PLANK POSE

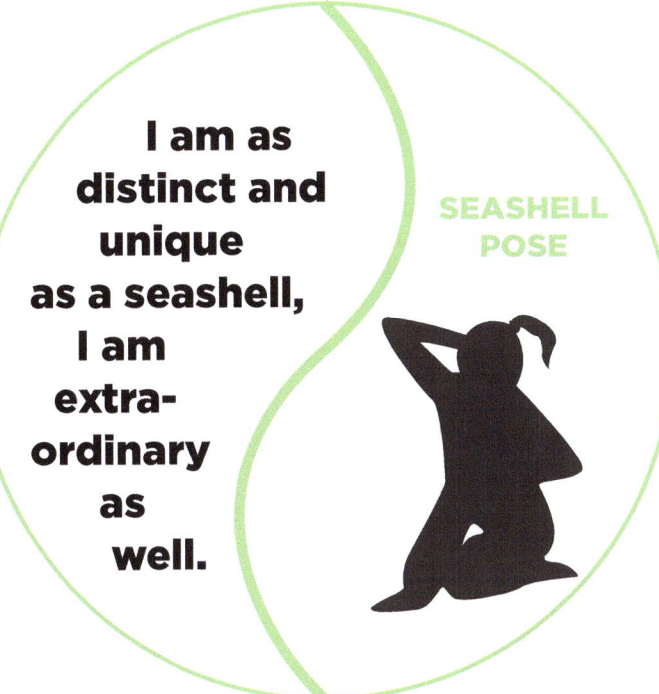

I am as distinct and unique as a seashell, I am extra-ordinary as well.

SEASHELL POSE

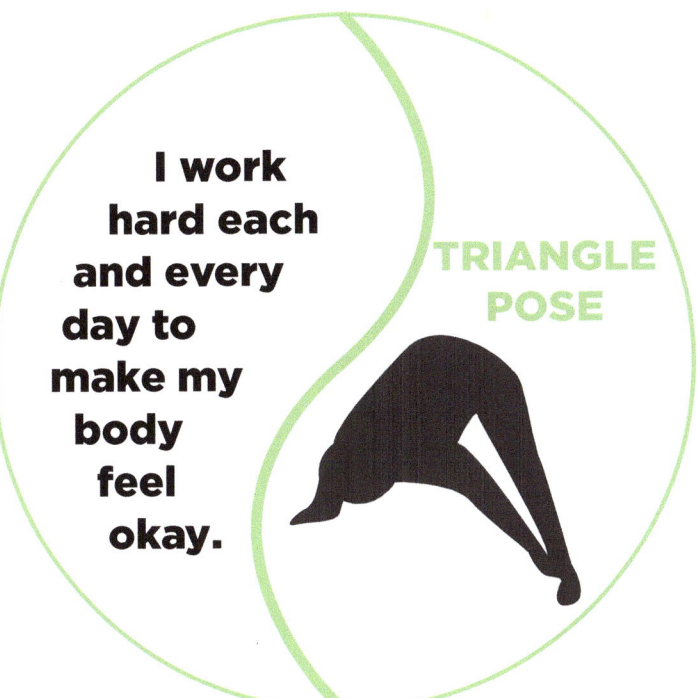

I work hard each and every day to make my body feel okay.

TRIANGLE POSE

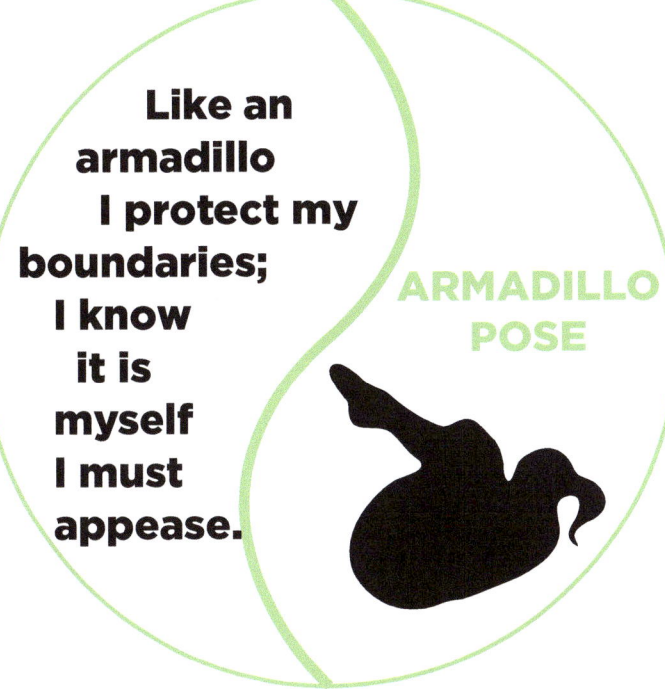

Like an armadillo I protect my boundaries; I know it is myself I must appease.

ARMADILLO POSE

I am
as strong
as a grizzly
bear and
I'm always
flexible
and
fair.

BEAR
POSE

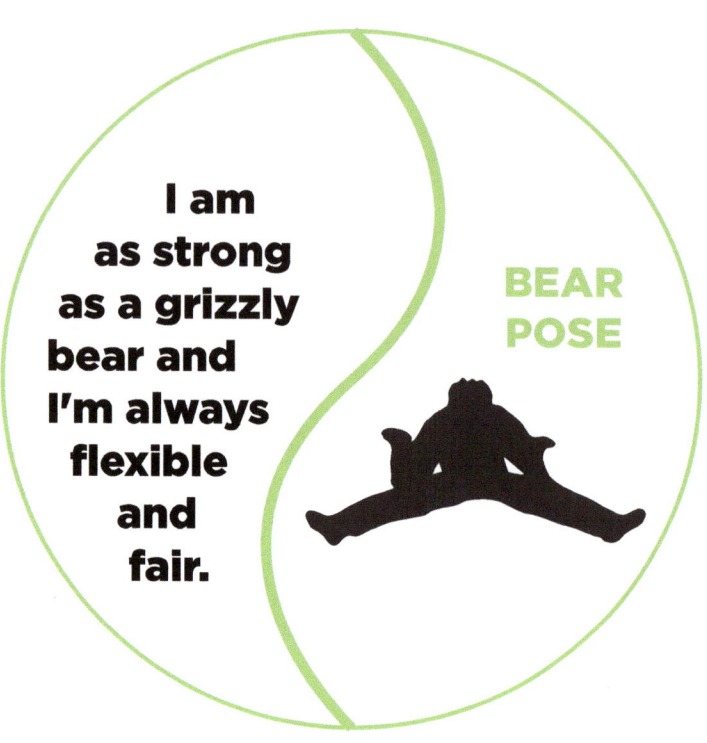

About the Author

Con reprehe ndellore exerspi enimolupta sanimo dolorerate accum diti unt rehenet erro mos et explitisque se erit lique rest repro digenderum vercimus ea volupta tinctiam quis ereptus molum invererrupta nus aliscii scidita diosseque quis idunti asitia volupta tibus, nusam lab in porepel estibus.

Eriae maio. Occabor ad magnihi lloritae pa voluptis aut quia doluptae se nus vent verrovidel illessi molentiuntem vel in reped mostis si re eium quid unt ea voluptae lati asinvelendit vent lab il maios eume nobit quiatiur, volori omnis evenditas doluptur, que eos eumquatem fugit lant unt vella sincto eum, voluptatur, que eici restota speribus voloribus vitatem laboraeste et aliquam eius magnat il magnime et modit asperias sa dolorrum estia nonsedi utem non nist eum quam quam quuntius, ute sed qui torro temquat quamus.

Ecab il in necae reptur, quos quis dolenis aut fugit fugitent lit es molorestium nobit et est vernat hil int.

Quid magnate mporepu daectem quatibus delia il ium, con recum, consequist, que doluptiates voluptatate elique qui dis ilibus dolor aut veliqui aut etusciis debit quam core provid enimagnam fugiatis preprepre plicae niminul litios aut quam, audandi scipist, quos aliam erum restium senis et, si dolorio idio tet, officil magnima gnimet harchit ecaborum vendel inctenem dolorem unt vid qui te esequod quos apero que dolorerchil ipiciet volupta vellesti tem hil ipsa volorrovit que vid maxima voluptis quid ut aut odicid mo occumqui conseque nis iur? Sae quossun discimincia sa solor mod ea dusae pelit, tem untur?

Bit erspero vitemodi consed qui dolorerum in perunt.

Aperepero conessincia que es nis ipsumquatem nos dolorerspel int mosa venientiat assumquo occat enim facea nimaiorempos anda con natet et aut quos aut officium, quam

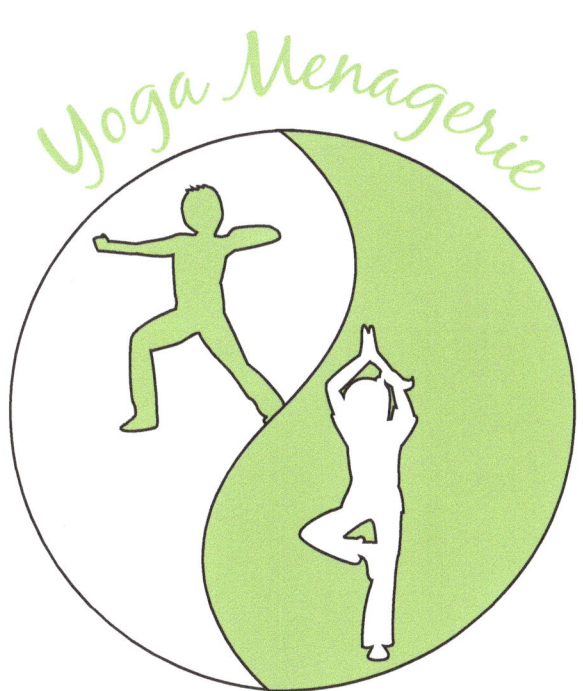

www.ingramcontent.com/pod-product-compliance
Lightning Source LLC
Chambersburg PA
CBHW050857180526
45159CB00007B/2701